For the Love of Gluten Free

Chef Joz

Copyright © 2025 Chef JoZ

All rights reserved worldwide.

No part of the book may be copied or changed in any format, sold, or used in a way other than what is outlined in this book, under any circumstances, without the prior written permission of the publisher.

Author: Chef Joz

Title: **For the Love of Gluten Free**

ISBN: 979-8-9995269-0-8 (Book)
ISBN: 979-8-9995269-1-5 (eBook)

DEDICATION

This book is dedicated to the people whose hearts and hands helped bring these recipes to life.

To **Jean Stevens,** my mother. Thank you for teaching me how to cook, for passing on all your knowledge, and for the example you set for me my entire life.

To **Brad Stewart,** my husband. Thank you for being a willing and enthusiastic taste-tester, and for the constant support you've given throughout this journey.

And to my three closest friends — **Deb, Rozi,** and **Renee**. Thank you for your encouragement, laughter, and friendship. Thank you for cheering this journey on from day one.

I LOVE you all,
Chef Joz

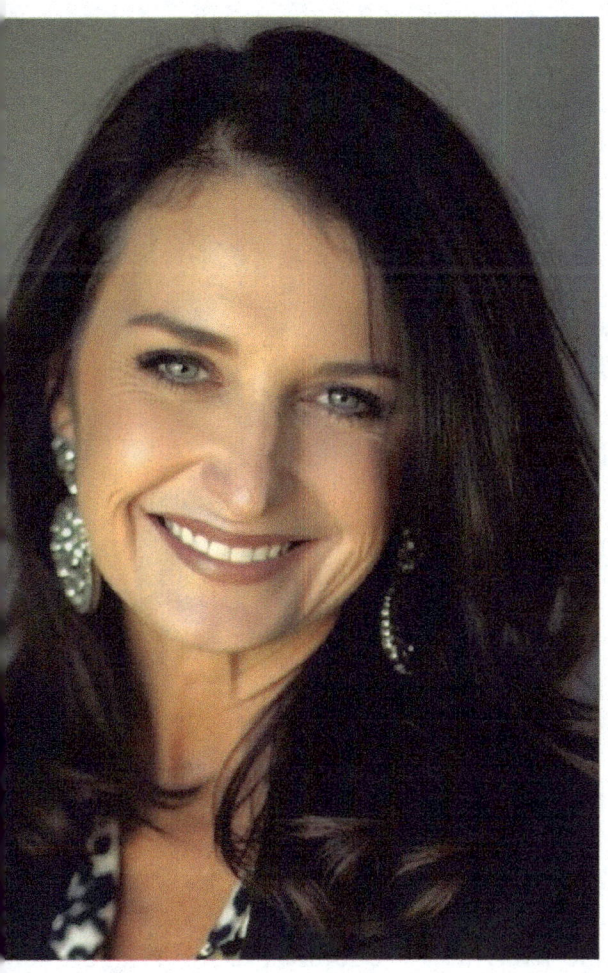

JOANIE IVY STEWART

Born and raised in Amarillo, Texas, Joanie Ivy Stewart has been perfecting her Gluten Free craft in the kitchen for over 20 years. A passionate cook with a love for creating meals that bring people together, Joanie's culinary journey is deeply rooted in her Southern heritage and enriched by her mother, who is also Gluten Free, and has been cooking Gluten Free for over 20 years. Her mother's wisdom and experiences have played a huge part in the success of Joanie's Gluten Free cooking.

When she's not in the kitchen, Joanie enjoys golfing with her husband Brad, spending quality time with her kids and grandkids, and exploring new destinations with friends. She splits her time between her home in Amarillo, Texas, where she also runs a successful business, and the serene countryside of Mt. Ulla, North Carolina.

Joanie's recipes reflect her life's joy— family, friends, and unforgettable flavors.

CONTENTS

Introductory 8

APPETIZERS, SAUCES, & DIPS 9
    JōZ Gluten Free Trail Mix 10
    JōZ Jalapeño Poppers 11
    JōZ Guacamole 12
    JōZ Queso Blanco 13
    Parmesan Zucchini Sticks 14
    Cheesy Green Chile Chicken Dip 15
    Pretzels Bites and Cheese Dip 16
    GF Ham & Cheese Puffs 18
    BBQ Bacon Wrapped Pineapple 19
    Charcuterie Board 19
    Fried Veggies 20
    Renee's Dip 21
    Rozi's Corn Dip 22
    Green Chile Enchilada Sauce 22
    JōZ Mexican Seasoning 23
    JōZ Honey Mustard 24

DESSERTS & SWEET BREADS 25
    GF Texas Chocolate Sheet Cake 26
    Chocolate Layered Cake 28
    Red Velvet Cake 30
    Blueberry Almond Cake w/ White Chocolate Frosting 32
    Cinnamon Crème Brulée 34
    Payday Fudge 35
    Layered Pie 36
    Key Lime Pie 37
    Chocolate Pie 38
    Buttermilk Pie (Lemon or Maple flavor) 39
    JōZ Cookie 40
    JōZ Chocolate Cookie 41
    Chocolate Chip Cookies 42
    Key Lime Cupcakes 43
    Strawberry Cupcakes 45
    Pumpkin Cupcakes or Muffins 46
    Mini Cheesecake & Fried Cheesecake Bites 47

    Fried Cheesecake Bites 48
    Blueberry Lime Bread 49
    Banana Chocolate Chip Bread 51
    JōZ Churro's 52

MAIN COURSES 53
    Beef Tips and Mashed Potatoes 54
    Brown Gravy 55
    Mashed Potatoes 55
    Baked Chicken and Shrimp Alfredo 56
    Grilled Chicken Fettuccine 58
    Chicken and Rice 60
    Gluten Free Pizza 61
    JōZ Chicken Tenders 63
    Baked Fish 64
    Fried Fish 65
    Shrimp Tacos 66
    JōZ's Chaunklas 67
    Deb and Seedie's Arizona Tacos 68
    Pigs In A Blanket 69
    Chicken Fried Steak Bites 70
    Steak Bites 71
    Spanish Rice 72
    Onion Rings 73
    Broccoli and Rice Casserole 74
    Santa Fe Soup 75
    Taco Soup 76

BREADS, PASTRIES & CRUST 77
    Corn Bread 78
    Puff Pastry 79
    JōZ Crescent Rolls 80
    JōZ Biscuits 81
    JōZ Pie Crust 82
    JōZ Graham Cracker Pie Crust 83
    JōZ Corn Tortilla 84

Products I Use In This Cookbook 85

*For the **Love** of **Gluten Free***

INTRODUCTORY

First off, I want to say **Thank You** for buying *For The Love of Gluten Free!* Whether you're new to gluten-free cooking or a seasoned pro, I'm thrilled to share this collection of recipes with you. Each dish has been crafted with love, tested in my own kitchen, and designed to make gluten-free living both delicious and simple.

A FEW IMPORTANT NOTES:

Recipes Videos Available Online

As a special bonus, every recipe in this cookbook is also available in video form on my website. Visit **chefjoz.com** and use the code **GF25** to access videos of the recipes where I walk you through how to prepare them, complete with my Chef JoZ tips and variations. As with everything else, Gluten Free cooking is always evolving and changing so keep checking the website for improvements and upgrades to these recipes and their ingredients.

SYMBOLS TO GUIDE YOU

To make navigating this cookbook even easier, I've included helpful symbols throughout the recipes:

- ***** : Indicates a special Chef JoZ tip located at the bottom of the recipe.
- **GF** : Indicates Gluten Free

You'll find these icons located next to the ingredients for each recipe.

YOU ARE MAKING A DIFFERENCE

Proceeds from the sale of this cookbook will go to support **The Agape Center** in Amarillo, Texas. **The Agape Center** is a peer-run mental health support hub which also provides transportation within the Amarillo area and serves as a welcoming space for individuals navigating mental health challenges.

FROM MY KITCHEN TO YOURS

I hope this cookbook inspires you to get creative in the kitchen and makes your gluten-free journey easier and more enjoyable. Thank you for allowing me to be a part of your meals. Happy cooking!

With gratitude,
"Chef JoZ"
Joanie Ivy Stewart

Appetizers, Sauces, & Dips

JōZ Gluten Free Trail Mix

INGREDIENTS

- 120 g Rice Chex
- 120 g Corn Chex
- 120 g GF pretzels*
- 100 g GF cheese cracker/puffs*
- 250 g mixed nuts
- 2.5 sticks of butter (melted/salted)
- 6 Tbsp Lea & Perrins Worcestershire Sauce
- 1.5 Tbsp Lawry's Seasoned Salt
- 1.5 tsp Garlic powder
- 1 tsp Chili powder
- 2 tsp Cayenne pepper*
- 1 Dash of paprika

1. Preheat oven to 350°F.
2. In a large mixing bowl add chex, pretzels, puffs, and nuts. Set aside.
3. In a medium size mixing bowl, melt butter, then add all seasoning and Worcestershire sauce and stir.
4. Pour over dry mixture in large bowl and gently stir with rubber spatula coating dry mixture with liquid mixture.
5. Take an extra-large sheet pan or 2 large sheet pans and pour mixture evenly on to pan/pans.
6. Bake for 15 minutes then gently stir mixture and rotate pan. Bake for an additional 15 minutes. Remove from oven and let cool! Enjoy

JōZ Tip: The Gluten Free pretzels can be a mixture of shapes. I recommend 2 different brands of cheese crackers.... Made Good and Simple Mills. See video for more details regarding ingredients. Cayenne pepper can be eliminated in this recipe if you do not like heat!

For the Love of Gluten Free

JōZ Jalapeño Poppers

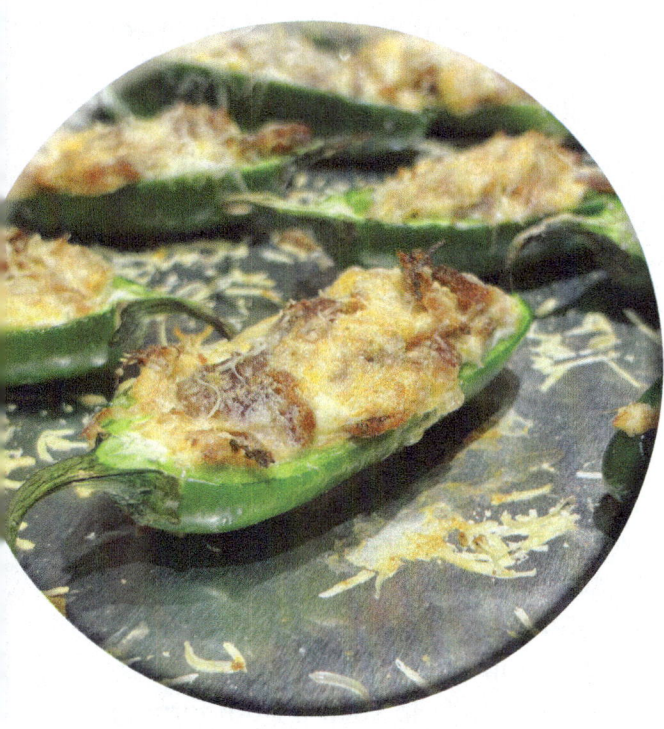

1. Line baking sheet with parchment paper or foil and spray with nonstick spray.
2. Preheat oven to 400°F.
3. Cut peppers in half, deseed, and remove the membranes. Rinse and set aside to dry.
4. In a large mixing bowl, add cream cheese, cheddar cheese, garlic powder, Lawry's seasoning, pulled pork, and bacon. Mix thoroughly.
5. Fill each ½ Pepper generously with mixture and place on baking sheet. Sprinkle lightly with fresh grated Parmesan Cheese if desired.
6. Cook for 20 mins and ENJOY!

JōZ Tip: Make sure your pulled pork and bacon are gluten free. DO NOT use pre-shredded cheese. When you are cutting the jalapenos in half DO NOT cut the stems off. This holds the goodness inside the pepper and keeps all your hard work from leaking out. Remember to wear gloves. 😊

INGREDIENTS

- 8-10 good size jalapeño peppers*
- 8 oz of cream cheese (softened)
- 2-4 oz fresh Cheddar cheese (shredded)
- 1 tsp garlic powder
- 1 tsp Lawry's seasoned salt
- 8-10 oz of cooked pulled pork
- 8 slices of cooked crispy bacon (chopped)
- 1 Tbsp freshly grated Parmesan Cheese (optional)

For the Love of Gluten Free

JōZ Guacamole

INGREDIENTS

4 medium avocados
Lime juice from 1 lime
1 tsp garlic salt
2 tsp Lawry's™ Seasoned Salt
2 small jalapeños
Onion (optional)
Diced Cherry tomatoes (optional)
Splash of jalapeño juice

1. Cut avocados in half and place seed to the side for later.
2. Taking each half of the avocado, scrape all the goodness into a large bowl.
3. Using a fork, mash avocados leaving small chunks.
4. Add lime juice, garlic salt, splash of jalapeño juice & Lawry's™ seasoned salt. Mix with fork until combined.
5. Cut jalapeños in half, deseed, and remove the membrane. Rince and chop these into small pieces and add to bowl. Add diced onions and diced tomatoes if you wish.
6. Fold gently until combined. Place the seeds in the bowl on top of the guacamole to help keep it from turning.
7. Serve with tortilla chips. YUM!

Jōz Tip: If you have leftovers, take some cling wrap and place it where it is touching the surface of the guacamole. Then cover with a lid.

JōZ Queso Blanco

INGREDIENTS

- 8 oz of fresh White Cheddar cheese (shredded)
- 4 oz cream cheese (room temperature)
- 8 oz Velveeta Queso Blanco cheese
- 8 oz fresh Pepper Jack cheese (shredded)
- 1 12 oz can evaporated milk
- 1 Tbsp butter
- 1-2 jalapenos seeded and chopped
- 4 oz Green Chilies*
- 1/2 tsp garlic salt
- 1/8 tsp cumin
- 1 pinch of cayenne
- ½ tsp salt
- 120-240 ml milk (warmed)

1. Using a medium size saucepan, melt butter, White Cheddar cheese, cream cheese, evaporated milk, and seasonings on **LOW** heat. CAREFUL NOT TO SCORCH.
2. Line your crockpot with a liner and set temperature to **LOW**.
3. Cut Velvetta into small squares and add to your crockpot. Pour green chilies over the top. Add your shredded Pepper Jack cheese and chopped jalapeños.
4. After your cheddar mixture has warmed and cheese has melted and is smooth, take and pour into crockpot. Gently stir.
5. Heat on low for 1-2 hours until smooth and hot. Add warm milk if queso is too thick.
6. Serve with chips or veggies.

Jōz Tip: I recommend using a good quality brand of cheese. **DO NOT** use pre-shredded cheese! See video for my recommendation for green chiles. This is a large batch which allows for leftovers. Reheat the necessary amount in sauce pan slowly adding milk to desired thinness.

For the Love of Gluten Free

Parmesan Zucchini Sticks

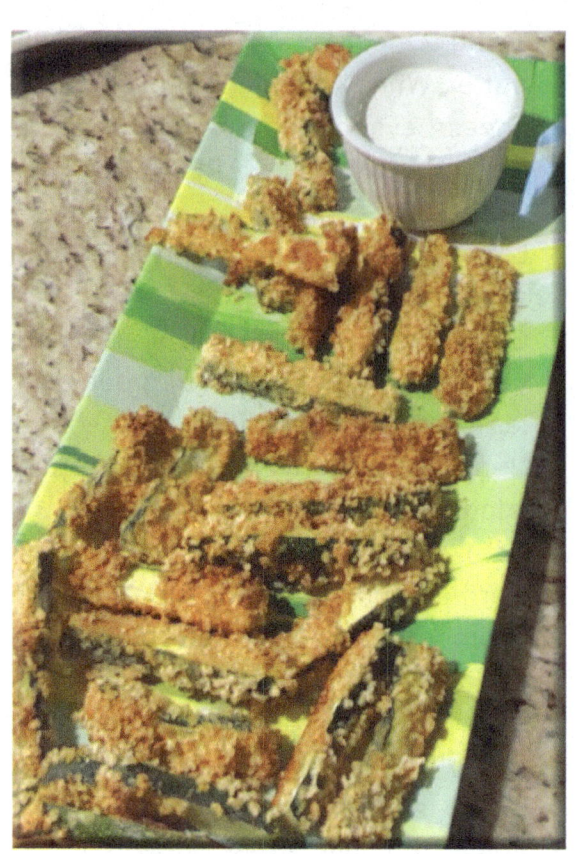

INGREDIENTS

2 medium zucchinis
½ cup GF Flour*
2 eggs
1 tsp Garlic powder
¼ tsp Paprika
¼ tsp Chili powder
½ tsp salt
1 Cup GF Breadcrumbs*
1 Cup Parmesan Cheese

1. Heat oven to 425° F.
2. Line a large baking sheet with parchment paper placing a wire rack on top. IMPORTANT: Spray wire rack with non-stick spray.
3. Slice ends off zucchini, then cut in half. Take each half and cut in half long ways. Take each half and cut into 3 equal long strips. You should have 24 slices. Each zucchini produces 12 slices. Set zucchini aside to dry. (I like to do this earlier in the day, because zucchini contains a lot of water)
4. Using a shallow dish, add flour and set aside.
5. Take a medium size bowl and place eggs in and slightly beat.
6. In another shallow dish (I like to use a large dish) place breadcrumbs, cheese, garlic, paprika, chili powder, and salt.
7. Take slice of zucchini and roll completely in flour, dip in egg mixture, then dip into bread crumb mixture. Place on wire rack and repeat with each slice.
8. Bake for 20-25 minutes. Enjoy with homemade Ranch dressing or sauce of your choice.

Jōz Tips: My suggestions on the best GF breadcrumbs are in the video! I use Bob's Red Mills GF Flour™.

Cheesy Green Chile Chicken Dip

INGREDIENTS

Approx 2 cups of cooked chicken (shredded)*
240 ml of chicken broth
8 oz cream cheese softened
160 g sour cream
60 ml Green Chile enchilada sauce (See recipe in cookbook) or your favorite brand
4 oz diced green chiles
2.0 oz Monterey Jack cheese shredded
2.0 oz Mozzarella cheese shredded
1 tsp salt
½ tsp black pepper

1. Heat oven to 375° F.
2. In a large mixing bowl, add cream cheese and sour cream and mix until smooth.
3. Add chicken broth and green enchilada sauce and mix with a large spoon until everything is combined. It should be a little soupy.
4. Add chicken, green chiles, cheeses, salt and pepper, and mix with a spoon until combined.
5. Pour mixture into a cast iron skillet or a casserole dish and spread evenly.
6. Bake for 20-30 minutes or until bubbling and starting to brown on top.
7. Serve with tortilla chips.

Jōz Tip: Using the homemade green chile enchilada sauce and a fresh boiled chicken makes a huge difference in this recipe. My recommendations on green chiles are in the video!

Pretzels Bites and Cheese Dip

INGREDIENTS

PRETZEL BITES

- 412 g of Gluten Free flour*
- 2 Tbsp brown sugar
- 1 tsp Salt
- 1 tsp baking powder
- 180 ml warm water 110°F degrees
- 1 pkg active dry yeast
- 1 Tbsp honey
- 140 ml warm milk
- 1 egg
- melted butter and coarse salt
- Baking soda bath (5-6 cups of water, ¼ cup of baking soda)

Gluten Free Beer Cheese dip

- 2 Tbsp butter
- 2 Tbsp Gluten Free Flour*
- 4 oz freshly shredded Monterrey Jack cheese
- 4 oz cream cheese softened
- 8 oz freshly shredded cheddar cheese
- 120+ ml beer* (optional)
- 180+ ml milk
- 60 ml heavy cream
- 2 tsp Dijon mustard
- ½ tsp garlic powder
- ½ tsp onion powder
- ¼ tsp cayenne
- 8 pieces of cooked bacon pieces (extra crispy)(optional)
- Salt and pepper to taste

1. In a large measuring cup mix water, yeast and honey and let set for 5 mins.
2. Using a stand mixing bowl whisk together flour, brown sugar, salt, & baking powder.
3. Pour water/yeast mixture, milk and egg over your dry ingredients and use the paddle attachment of the stand mixer beat on medium speed for about 4 minutes. Dough is sticky!
4. Transfer dough on to a liberally floured work surface and knead dough until it becomes smooth.
5. Place dough in a lightly greased bowl, cover and allow it to rise for approximately 1 hour. Almost double in size.
6. Preheat the oven to 425°F and line a large baking sheet with parchment paper.
7. Using a large pot, start your baking soda bath by bringing water to boil. (don't add soda yet)
8. Transfer the dough to a slightly floured surface and work until a ball of dough is formed adding flour as needed. Divide into 6-8 equally sections. Take one section and patiently work with rolling it out into a "rope" about an inch thick.
9. Take a sharp knife and cut dough into 1.5-inch-long pieces. Repeat until you have used all the dough.

10. By this time, your water should be boiling. Add soda and as soon as the foam subsides, add about 8-10 bites to the water and boil for 20 seconds. Using a slotted spoon, remove bites and place them on baking sheet lined with parchment paper. Repeat until all bites are done.
11. Place the bites in oven and cook 6-8 minutes, until golden brown. Remove from oven.
12. Using a pastry brush, brush each bite with melted butter and sprinkle with coarse salt.

CHEESE DIP
(I like to start this while dough is rising)

1. Melt butter in a large saucepan on medium high heat. Add flour and whisking continually for about 2 minutes.
2. Add milk, heavy cream, beer, and seasonings stir constantly.
3. Add cheese and turn down to low. Cook slowly, stirring occasionally to make sure cheese does not stick.
4. As cheese melts, you can add bacon bites at this time.
5. Add salt and pepper to taste.
6. Remove from heat and serve warm with pretzel bites. (I like to transfer cheese dip to a small mini crockpot and keep on warm)

Jōz Tip: I use Cup 4 Cup™ GF flour. Make sure you use a Gluten Free Beer or Nonalcoholic Gluten Free Beer, but if you choose not to use beer, just replace the liquid with milk. This cheese dip tends to lean on the thick side so don't be afraid to add more liquid. 😊

GF Ham & Cheese Puffs

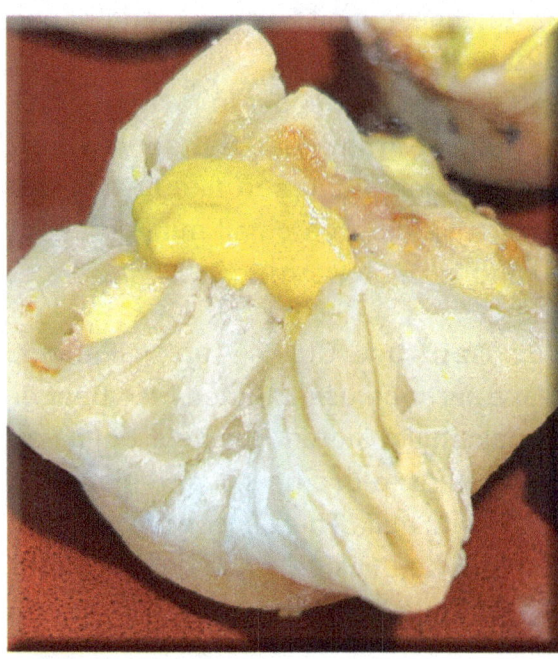

INGREDIENTS

- 1 recipe of JōZ puff pastry (recipe in cookbook)
- 5 - 6 oz of finely chopped ham
- 4-5 oz of fresh Pepper Jack or Colby Jack cheese (shredded)
- 2 eggs
- 1 tsp salt
- ½ tsp ground mustard
- ½ tsp pepper
- ¼ tsp garlic salt
- 1 Egg wash

1. Preheat oven to 410°F.
2. Spray **EVERY OTHER** hole in a mini muffing pan with nonstick spray.
3. Roll out JōZ puff pastry in a large rectangle.
4. Using a pizza cutter, cut squares in an approximate size of 3x3" and place on top of holes that have been sprayed with nonstick spray.
5. Using a medium bowl, mix chopped ham, cheese, eggs, and seasonings until combined.
6. Using a small scoop, fill each square with ham and cheese mixture.
7. Pull up each corner of dough and pinch together. I like to brush the corners with a little egg wash to help them stick and hold in place while baking.
8. Bake for approximately 12-15 minutes. Serve while warm! I love to dip them in mustard!

JōZ Tip: Make sure you follow the puff pastry recipe. The video helps tremendously with this recipe. **DO NOT** use pre-shredded cheese!

BBQ Bacon Wrapped Pineapple

INGREDIENTS

1 Can of pineapple chunks (drained)
1 pkg of bacon (regular)
Barbeque sauce*
toothpicks

1. Preheat oven to 400°F.
2. Line cookie sheet with foil and spray with nonstick spray.
3. Cut bacon in half and wrap bacon around a pineapple chunk and secure with a toothpick. Place it on cookie sheet. Continue until you have wrapped all the pineapple chunks.
4. Using a brush, baste SLIGHTLY with your favorite BBQ sauce. Cook for approximately 20 mins and remove from oven and baste again with BBQ sauce. Increase temperature to 425° and cook another 5-10 mins. Remove from the oven and enjoy!

JōZ Tip: I love to use Sweet Baby Rays™ Original BBQ Sauce. It is gluten free. Also, I like to use regular bacon and not thick cut. It cooks more evenly.

Charcuterie Board

Meats
Cheese
Fruits
Veggies
Assorted nuts
Assorted candies

Bacon wrapped pineapple*
Prosciutto wrapped pickle*
Caprese Skewers*
pretzel mini dogs*

JōZ Tip: Watch VIDEO

For the Love of Gluten Free

Fried Veggies

INGREDIENTS

60 g GF Flour*
300 ml buttermilk
2 extra large eggs
200 g GF breadcrumbs*
8 Tbsp rice flour
5 Tbsp corn starch
1 tsp baking powder
1 tsp garlic salt
2 tsp salt
1 tsp black pepper
1 tsp Slap Ya Mama™ seasoning
2 large jalapeños
1 large zucchini
1 large squash
Your favorite dipping sauce

1. Cut ends off jalapeños, squash, and zucchini. Cut stem off jalapeños then cut in half long ways and deseed each side. Cut each half in 3 long strips. You should have 12 long slices.
2. Take zucchini or squash and cut in half. Take each half and cut in half long ways. Take each half and cut into 3 equal long strips. You should have 12 long slices.
3. In a large zip baggie, place your GF Flour, sliced jalapenos, zucchini, and squash and gently shake to coat all veggies.
4. At this time start heating vegetable oil in a large skillet or deep fryer to 375°F.
5. In a medium bowl, whisk buttermilk and eggs together and set aside.
6. In a large mixing bowl, combine breadcrumbs, rice flour, corn starch, soda, and seasonings. Set aside.
7. Take each flour coated veggie and dip into the buttermilk/egg mixture and then into the bread crumb mixture. Place coated veggies into hot oil and cook until each side is crispy and golden brown.
8. Serve with homemade ranch dressing.

JōZ Tip: I use King Arthur™ GF flour for this recipe. It produces a crispier coating. Also, feel free to use other veggies such as mushrooms, pickles, or asparagus. My suggestions on the best GF breadcrumbs are in the video!

Renee's Dip

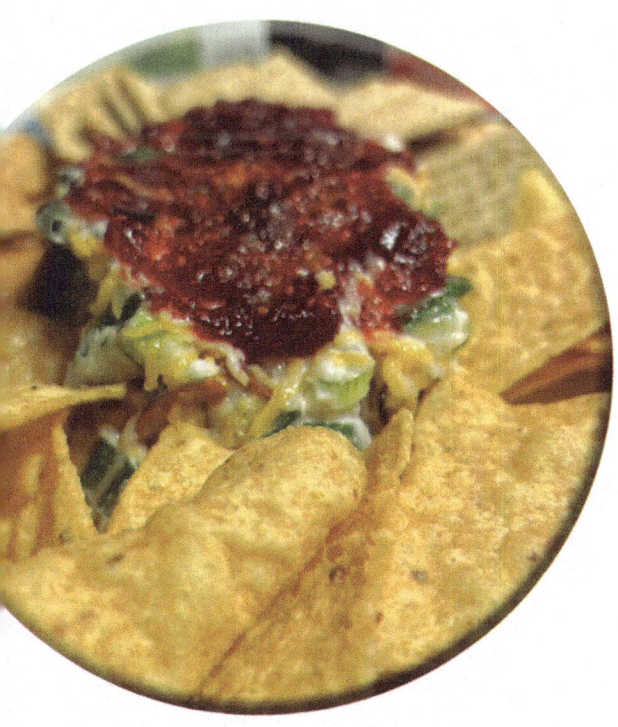

INGREDIENTS

- 1 Cup mayonnaise
- 1 Cup toasted sliced almonds
- 1 Cup shredded Cheddar cheese*
- 1/2 Cup chopped green onion
- 8 slices of bacon cooked to crispy (optional)
- Plum or Raspberry jam (or your favorite)

1. Cook 8 slices of bacon to crispy and set aside to cool.
2. Heat a large skillet to medium high, pour sliced almonds into the skillet and constantly stir until nice and toasted. DO NOT WALK AWAY.
3. In a large bowl, add mayonnaise and toasted almonds, then add in cheese, green onions, and bacon if desired.
4. Place dip in the refrigerator to cool for at least an hour.
5. When ready to serve, remove dip from the refrigerator and spread on a platter. Spread a thin layer of your favorite jam over the top and serve with tortilla chips or crackers.

Renee Tip: Renee recommends using pre-shredded cheese. Make sure you watch the video so you can meet Renee!

Rozi's Corn Dip

INGREDIENTS

- 1 can yellow and white corn (Drained)
- 2 cans Mexican corn (Drained)
- 2 cups of shredded cheese
- 1 cup mayonnaise
- 1 cup sour cream
- ½ cup green onion chopped
- 1-2 large jalapeños chopped
- 1-2 tsp Holy Voodoo™ Seasoning

1. In a large mixing bowl, mix all ingredients except the seasoning until well combined. Add seasoning until you reach desired taste. Serve with tortilla chips.

Rozi Tip: Rozi suggests making sure you refrigerate this dip overnight if possible. Make sure you watch the video so you can meet Rozi!

Green Chile Enchilada Sauce

INGREDIENTS

- 2 Tbsp canola oil divided
- 50 g chopped onions
- 1 extra-large jalapeño
- 3 garlic cloves chopped
- 10 oz green chiles*
- 1 tsp vinegar
- 1 tsp salt
- 1 tsp cumin
- 16 g cornstarch
- 240 ml chicken or vegetable

1. In a medium saucepan or skillet, sauté onions and jalapeños in canola oil for approximately three minutes or until onions look translucent.
2. Add garlic and cook for another minute or so.
3. Add mixture to food processor or blender (be careful, it's hot). Add green chiles, salt, cumin, and vinegar and blend to a nice smooth mixture.
4. Pour mixture back into pan.
5. In a small bowl, mix corn starch and chicken stock or broth until they are combined. Add these to your pan and cook for 5-8 mins.
6. This yumminess is ready!

JōZ Tip: Use fresh green chiles if possible. Also, store the remaining sauce in the refrigerator for up to 3-4 days.

For the Love of Gluten Free

JōZ Mexican seasoning

INGREDIENTS

- 2 Tbsp Chili Powder
- 1 Tbsp Paprika
- 1 Tbsp Cumin
- 1 tsp Garlic Powder
- 2 tsp Onion Powder
- 1 tsp dried oregano
- 1 tsp salt
- ¼ tsp ground black pepper
- ½ tsp cayenne pepper
- ½ tsp red pepper

Mix all ingredients together and use when making tacos, enchiladas, or any recipe that calls for taco seasoning.

JōZ Honey Mustard

INGREDIENTS

150 g of mayonnaise (your favorite brand)
3 Tbsp Mustard
1 tsp Dijon Mustard
2 tsp apple cider vinegar
85 g of honey
¼ tsp salt
¼ tsp paprika
¼ tsp garlic powder
pinch of cayenne pepper

Mix all ingredients in a medium bowl until smooth. Refrigerate for about 30 minutes before serving.

JōZ Tip: I love to use a Hot Honey. See video for my favorite brand.

DESSERTS & SWEET BREADS

GF Texas Chocolate Sheet Cake

CAKE INGREDIENTS

300 g GF Flour*
400 g sugar
1 tsp baking powder
1 tsp soda
½ tsp salt
2 sticks of butter
30 g unsweetened cocoa powder
10 g unsweetened dark cocoa powder
240 ml water
120 ml buttermilk (room temp)
30 g sour cream (room temp)
2 egg (room temp)
1 tsp vanilla
1 tsp cinnamon

FROSTING INGREDIENTS

1 stick of butter
15 g unsweetened cocoa powder
5 g unsweetened dark cocoa powder
1-3 TBSP Half and Half or Heavy Cream
3-4 cups of Powdered sugar
1 tsp Vanilla
Nuts (optional)

1. Preheat oven to 375° F.
2. Grease a 15x10 sheet cake pan (jelly roll pan) and set aside.
3. Using a medium-sized saucepan, bring to a low boil your butter, cocoa, and water. Remove from heat and set aside.
4. In a large mixing bowl, sift together your flour, sugar, baking powder, soda, and salt.
5. In a small bowl, whisk your buttermilk, sour cream, and egg together.
6. Pour your chocolate mixture into your dry mixture and stir with large spoon until combined. Pour in buttermilk mixture and stir until combined.
7. Add vanilla and cinnamon and stir until the batter is completely smooth. **DO NOT USE A MIXER**.
8. Pour into sheet pan and cook for approximately 20 minutes or until a toothpick is inserted into the center of cake and comes out clean. **DO NOT OVERCOOK!**

WHILE CAKE IS COOKING PREPARE YOUR FROSTING.

1. In a microwave safe bowl, heat butter and cocoa until melted.
2. Add powdered sugar and alternate with a heavy cream a little at a time until you reach desired taste.
3. Add vanilla and beat for about 2 minutes.
4. Spread over cake as soon as you remove cake from oven.
5. **Eat morning, afternoon and for a midnight snack!**

JōZ Tip: I use Bob's Red Mill™ Gluten Free Baking Flour. The frosting for this cake does NOT have to be thick… I like it to be nice and smooth about the consistency of a pudding, and I just pour it over the hot cake. I think this is what makes the "Texas sheet cake".

Chocolate Layered Cake

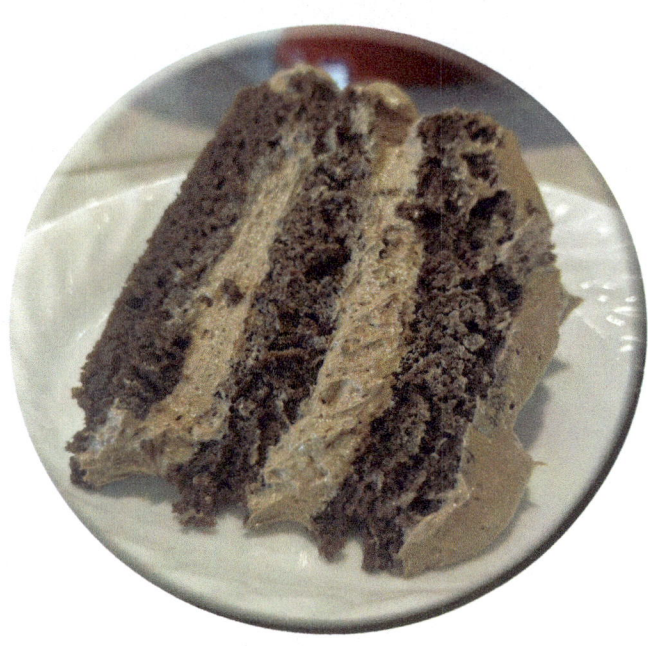

CAKE INGREDIENTS

285 g GF Flour*
200 g white sugar
1 tsp salt
1 tsp baking powder
2 sticks salted butter
240 ml water
30 g unsweetened cocoa powder
10 g unsweetened dark cocoa powder
2 eggs (room temp)
192 g dark brown sugar
½ tsp baking soda
1 tsp vinegar
120 g sour cream (full fat)
2 Tbsp milk (room temp)

CHOCOLATE FROSTING INGREDIENTS

3 sticks of unsalted butter
20 g cocoa
10 g extra dark cocoa
5-6 cups of powdered sugar
1 vanilla
150-180 ml heavy cream

CAKE

1. Heat oven to 350°F.
2. Line 3 8-inch round cake pans with parchment paper and spray sides with nonstick spray.
3. In a medium-sized saucepan, bring to a low boil butter, cocoa, and water. Remove from heat and set aside.
4. In a large mixing bowl, sift flour, white sugar, baking powder, and salt together and set aside.
5. In a small mixing bowl, whisk 2 eggs and brown sugar until nice and creamy.
6. Pour liquid chocolate mixture into your flour mixture. Mix with large spoon until combined. Next, pour butter mixture and brown sugar/egg mixture into batter and stir until smooth.

7. In a small bowl, mix milk with sour cream and add to mixture.
8. In a small measuring cup or small dish mix vinegar and soda. It will foam so no worries...you are now a chemist. 😉 Pour into batter and stir until completely smooth.
9. Add vanilla and stir till smooth.
10. Let batter rest for about 10 mins.
11. Using your scale, pour batter equally into each pan. Bake for approximately 20-25 minutes until toothpick is inserted into middle and comes out clean. **DO NOT OVER COOK**. Let cake cool completely before frosting.

FROSTING

1. Beat butter in a stand mixer for 6 minutes.
2. Sift together cocoa and powdered sugar and slowly add into mixer alternately with heavy cream.
3. Add vanilla and beat until desired thickness.
4. Frost Cake.

👨‍🍳 **JōZ Tip:** I use Bob's Red Mill ™ Gluten Free Baking Flour. Make sure you use a large spoon and not a mixer to mix your cake batter. Use a stand mixer for the frosting. This cake is super rich but so yummy!

Red Velvet Cake

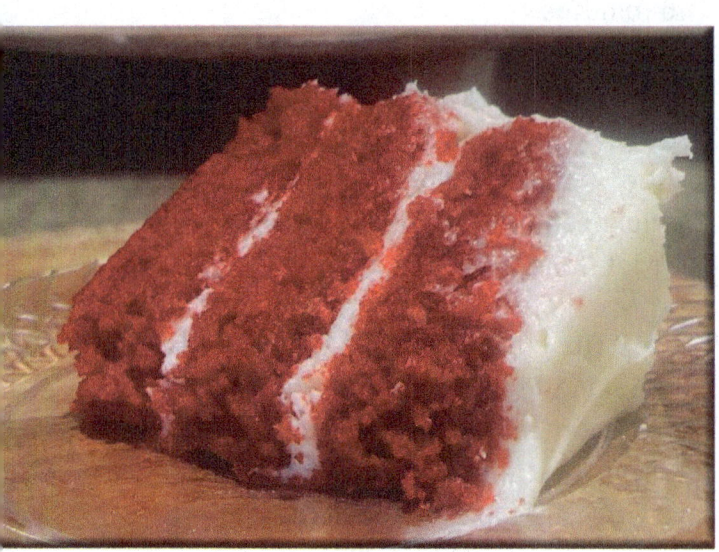

CAKE INGREDIENTS

4 Tbsp butter
240 ml canola oil
350 g white sugar
2 extra large eggs
1 tsp vanilla
red food coloring
285 g GF flour*
1 tsp salt
1 tsp baking powder
15 g unsweetened cocoa powder
240 ml buttermilk (room temp)
60 g sour cream (room temp)
½ tsp baking soda
2 tsp vinegar

CREAM CHEESE FROSTING INGREDIENTS

2 sticks of unsalted butter (softened)
8 oz block of cream cheese (softened)
4-6 cups of powdered sugar
2-4 Tbsp heavy whipping cream
1 tsp vanilla

CAKE

1. Preheat oven to 350°F.
2. Line three, 8-inch round cake pans **OR** four 6-inch round cake pans with parchment paper and spray sides with nonstick spray.
3. Using a stand mixer, beat butter on med-high for 2 minutes. Turn the speed to low and slowly add oil and mix for another minute. Add white sugar and beat until smooth and fluffy. Add egg one at a time until well combined. Add vanilla and red food coloring. (Add as much or as little as you want for desired color. I talk more about this in video.)
4. In a separate medium bowl, sift together flour, cocoa, salt and baking powder.
5. In small bowl, mix buttermilk and sour cream until smooth.

6. Add ½ of flour mixture to butter/oil mixture and stir with a spoon. (NOT MIXER) Add ½ of buttermilk/sour cream and continue to mix until mostly combined. Add remaining flour mixture and stir until combined and finally add remaining buttermilk/sour cream and stir until nice and smooth.
7. Lastly, in a small measuring cup or small dish, mix vinegar and soda. Add this to batter and stir until the batter is nice and smooth. Let batter rest for about 10 mins. Using your scale, pour batter equally into each pan. Bake for approximately 20-25 minutes until a toothpick is inserted into middle and comes out clean. DO NOT OVER COOK.

FROSTING

1. Using a stand mixer, whip butter on high for 5 minutes.
2. Add 2 oz of cream cheese at a time until well combined. Beat on high for 2-3 minutes.
3. Add powdered sugar slowly into mixer alternating with heavy cream. Add vanilla and beat until desired thickness.
4. Frost Cake.

JōZ Tip: I use Bob's Red Mill™ Gluten Free Baking Flour. Make sure you use a large spoon and not a mixer to mix the cake batter. Use a stand mixer for the frosting.

Blueberry Almond Cake w/ White Chocolate Frosting

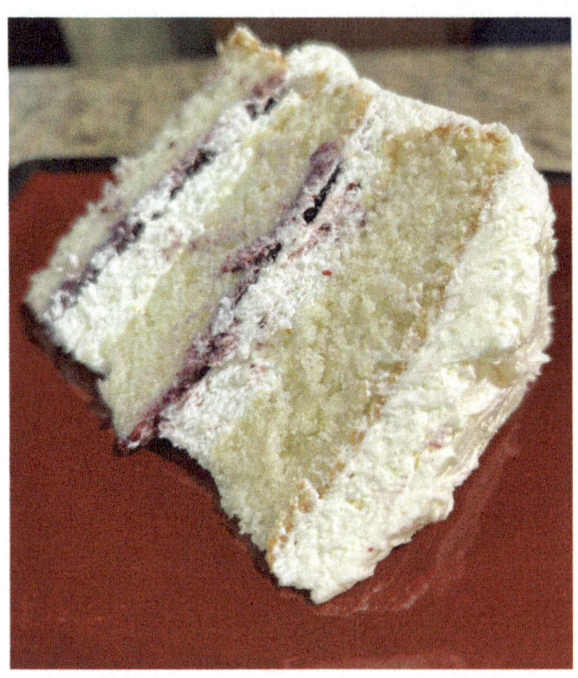

CAKE INGREDIENTS

327 g GF flour*
1 Tbsp baking powder
1 tsp salt
6 Tbsp unsalted butter (softened)
150 ml canola oil
400 g sugar
1 Tbsp almond extract
1 tsp vanilla
240 ml whole milk (room temperature)
30 g sour cream
6 egg whites

BLUEBERRY FILLING INGREDIENTS

225 g fresh blueberries rinsed
1 Tbsp water
4 Tbsp sugar
zest from 1 orange
juice from ½ orange

FROSTING INGREDIENTS

6 egg whites
300 g sugar
3 sticks of unsalted butter (room temp)
140-150 g white chocolate chips/wafers
1 tsp canola oil
1 tsp vanilla

BLUEBERRY FILLING

1. In a small saucepan, bring blueberries, water, sugar, zest, and juice from orange to a low boil. Turn heat down to low and let simmer for 20 minutes. Set aside and let completely cool.

CAKE

1. Preheat oven to 350°F.
2. Line three, 9-inch cake pans with parchment paper. Spray sides lightly with non-stick spray.

3. Whisk together flour, salt and baking powder in a medium bowl. Set it aside.
4. Using a stand mixer, beat butter for 3 minutes. Slowly pour in oil. Slowly pour in sugar and whip until light and fluffy. Set it aside.
5. Mix milk and sour cream in a separate measuring cup. Set it aside.
6. Beat egg whites in a medium mixing bowl until you reach medium/stiff peak. Set aside.
7. With a large spoon stir in 1/3 of flour mixture and 1/3 of milk mixture to your butter/oil/sugar mixture. Add another 1/3 of each and stir until combined. Add the final 1/3 of each and stir until combined.
8. Stir in almond flavor and vanilla.
8. Fold in egg whites until batter is completely combined and smooth.
9. Pour equal amounts of batter into the three, 9-inch round cake pans. Cook for approximately 20 mins or until a toothpick is inserted into center of cake and comes out clean. Let cool for about 5 mins in pan, then remove from pan. Let cake cool completely.

FROSTING

1. Using a large boiler, fill with 1-2 inches of water. Place your stand mixing bowl in boiler making sure the water is not touching bottom of mixing bowl.
2. Turn heat to medium-high and add egg whites and sugar. Whisk until mixture reaches 150-160° F. Remove from heat and let cool for about 2-3 mins.
3. Using your whisk attachment, beat on medium-high until stiff peak forms. Allow to cool completely.
4. Using a microwave safe bowl, add white chocolate chips and oil. Heat in microwave starting with 30 second intervals stirring in between until completely melted. Set aside.
5. Change to paddle attachment and turn on low. Slowly add 1 Tbsp of butter at a time making sure each slice is mixed in before adding the next. Continue until all butter is added.
6. Add the melted white chocolate and turn on high and beat for 5-10 minutes or until the frosting becomes nice and fluffy. 😊 (That's just the best description)

CAKE ASSEMBLY

1. Place the first cake on a serving plater or turn table. Spread ½ blueberry filling on top of cake and top with frosting.
2. Repeat with second cake.
3. Place final layer of cake on top and frost as desired.

JōZ Tip: I use Bob's Red Mill™ Gluten Free Baking Flour. The video is extremely helpful with this recipe. Especially the frosting!!! Also, for the love of desserts, do not throw out your egg yolks. Let us make some Crème Brulée.

For the Love of Gluten Free

Cinnamon Crème Brulée

INGREDIENTS

- 1 Quart heavy cream
- 1 tsp of vanilla paste
- 2 Cinnamon sticks
- 10 large egg yolks
- 200 g superfine granulated sugar, (DIVIDED) plus extra for caramelizing
- ½ tsp of salt

1. Preheat the oven to 300 F.
2. In a medium saucepan over medium low heat, combine the heavy cream, 100 g of sugar, and cinnamon stick. Cook until it starts to simmer or barely bubble, stirring constantly. Remove from heat and let sit and come to room temperature. Approximately 30 mins.
3. In a medium bowl, whisk the egg yolks, 100 g of sugar, vanilla paste and salt until smooth.
4. Remove the cinnamon sticks from the cream mixture and add the cream mixture to the egg yolks.
5. Whisk completely. I like to pour liquid through a super fine strainer or fine mesh sieve before I pour into ramekins.
6. Pour mixture into 8 ramekins.
7. Carefully place the ramekins in a deep baking dish and set the dish in the oven.
8. Slowly add hot water into the baking dish until water level reaches about ½ up the ramekins, careful not to splash on the custards.
9. Bake the custards until just set in the middle, for approximately 45 minutes.
10. Carefully remove from the oven let cool.
11. Refrigerate overnight.
12. Just before serving, sprinkle about a tsp of sugar on top of each ramekin. Use a kitchen torch or oven broiler to brown the tops. Sprinkle on the cinnamon. Serve.

JōZ Tip: It is very important to use superfine sugar. Don't let this recipe intimidate you! The video is a big help for this recipe.

Payday Fudge

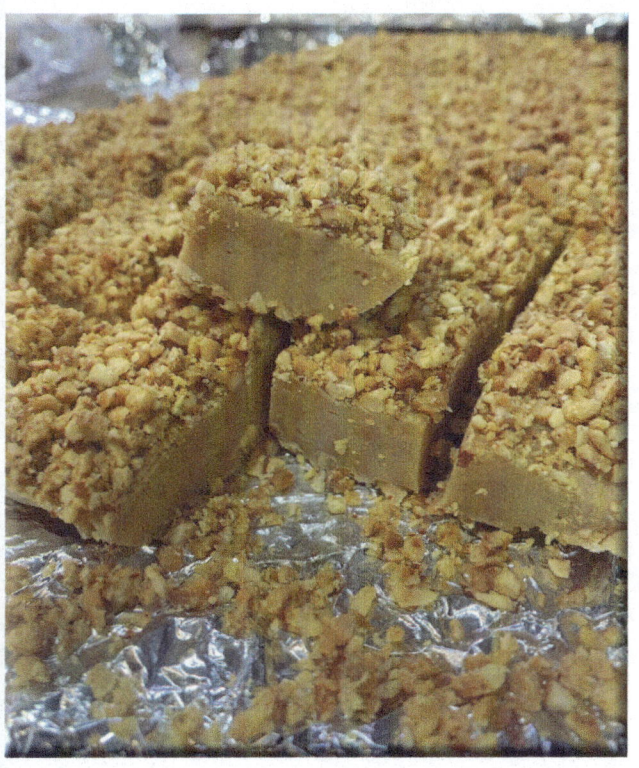

1. Line a 9x13 pan with foil and spray lightly with nonstick spray.
2. In a food processer, slightly grind the honey roasted peanuts. Sprinkle approximately ½ of these into bottom of pan.
3. In a large boiler, mix all other ingredients on low heat until the mixture is melted and smooth. Poor mixture over peanuts. Sprinkle the remaining peanuts over the top.
4. Refrigerate for at least 2 hours and cut into bars.

Kathleen Hill's Tip: Share with all your friends.

INGREDIENTS

4 cups of Honey Roasted Peanuts
1 can of Eagle Brand™
   (sweetened condensed milk)
16 oz pkg miniature marshmallows
10 oz pkg Peanut Butter chips
1 stick of butter
132 g peanut butter

Layered Pie

INGREDIENTS

- 1 JōZ GF Graham Cracker Crust recipe (Recipe in cookbook)
- 8 oz cream cheese (softened)
- 115 g powdered sugar
- 720 ml heavy whipping cream (divided)
- 2 Tbsp powdered sugar
- 1 Extra large spoon full of marshmallow cream (melted and cooled)
- 1 tsp vanilla
- 5 oz box of chocolate instant pudding
- 3 oz box of butterscotch instant pudding
- 5 cups of cold milk (DIVIDED)

1. Preheat oven to 350°F.
2. Prepare JōZ Graham Cracker Crust as directed.
3. Pour graham cracker mixture into a 9x13 dish and, using a fork, pat mixture evenly over bottom of pan. Cook for approximately 5 minutes. Place dish in the refrigerator to cool.
4. In a mixing bowl with a handheld mixer, beat heavy cream and 2 Tbsp of powdered sugar until you reach a stiff peak. Place bowl in refrigerator to stay cold.
5. In medium mixing bowl beat cream cheese and 115 g powdered sugar with a hand mixer until smooth.
6. Take heavy cream from the refrigerator and fold it into cream cheese mixture with a spoon.
7. Remove 9x13 dish out of the refrigerator and spread cream cheese mixture **gently** over graham cracker crust. Place back into refrigerator to chill.
8. Prepare chocolate pudding as directed on box. Remove pan from refrigerator and pour pudding over top of cream cheese mixture. Place back in the refrigerator.
9. Prepare butterscotch pudding as directed on box. Pour over top of chocolate pudding. Place dish back in the refrigerator.
10. In a cold mixing bowl, beat 480 ml of heavy cream, 1 tsp vanilla, and marshmallow cream with handheld mixer to a stiff peak. Spread over top of butterscotch pudding and refrigerate for at least 4 hours. Decorate if desired.

JōZ Tip: If possible, refrigerate this pie overnight… It just tastes better.

Key Lime Pie

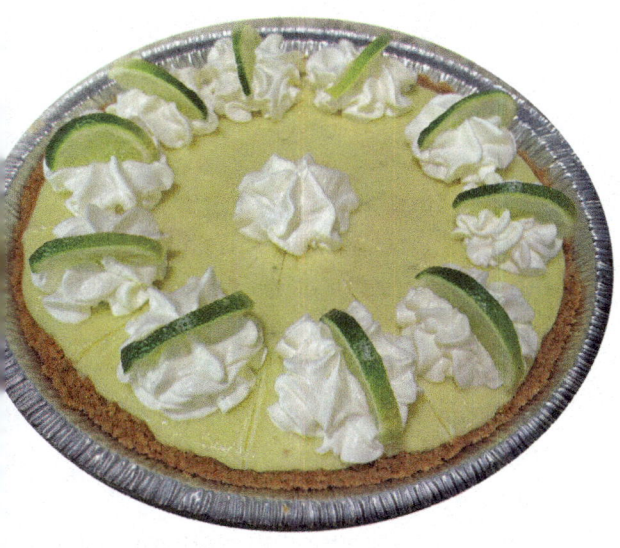

INGREDIENTS

- 1 JōZ GF Graham Cracker Crust recipe (Recipe in cookbook)
- 2 cans sweetened condensed milk (I love Eagle™ Brand)
- 120 g sour cream
- 2 egg yolks
- Zest from limes
- 180 ml key lime juice
- 2 drops lime oil*
- 1 green food coloring (optional)

1. Preheat oven to 350°F.
2. Prepare JōZ Graham Cracker Crust as directed. Using a fork, spread crumbs into an 8-inch pie dish.
3. Place in oven and bake for approximately 5 mins. Set aside to cool.
4. In a large mixing bowl, whip sweetened milk and sour cream on medium high speed until smooth.
5. Turn speed down to low and add egg yolks one at a time until combined.
6. Add in lime zest, lime juice, and lime oil and continue to beat on low until combined.
7. I like to add a couple of drops of green food coloring, but this is optional.
8. Pour filling over graham cracker crust and place back in the oven and cook for roughly 15 minutes or until center is jiggly. **DO NOT OVER COOK**.
9. Remove from oven and let cool. Refrigerate for at least 3 hours. Serve with homemade whipping cream! YUM

JōZ Tip: I like to use Young Living™ lime oil. Do not overbeat the mixture once you have added the egg yolks.

For the Love of Gluten Free

Chocolate Pie

INGREDIENTS

- 1 JōZ Pie Crust (Recipe in cookbook)
- 200 g sugar
- 32 g cornstarch
- 15 g cocoa powder
- 5 g dark cocoa powder
- ½ tsp salt
- 350 ml milk
- 125 ml evaporated milk
- 4 egg yolks (room temp)
- 2 Tbsp butter
- 1 tsp vanilla
- 5 egg whites (room temp)
- ¼ tsp cream of tarter
- 50 g of sugar

1. Prepare JōZ Pie Crust and blind bake as directed. Set aside to cool.
2. Using 2 small bowls, separate egg yolks and whites. MAKE SURE EGGS ARE ROOM TEMPERATURE.
3. In medium size boiler, whisk together sugar, cornstarch, cocoas, and salt. Turn heat to medium and whisk in milks. Continue to whisk until mixture starts to boil and continue to whisk for another minute or so. Remove from heat.
4. Using a spoon, take a little of the mixture and add to your egg yolks and stir. Continue to do this until you have tempered the eggs.
5. Add mixture back into the chocolate filling. Place back on medium heat and whisk for 3-4 minutes. The filling will start to be nice and thick.
6. Remove from heat and add butter and vanilla and stir until combined.
7. Poor filling into pie crust.
8. Preheat oven to 325°F
9. While the pie is cooling, add your egg whites and tarter to a stand mixer bowl and beat on medium high till soft peak forms. About 1-2 minutes.
10. Turn speed down to low and slowly add sugar. Turn speed back up to medium high and beat until a stiff peak is formed.
11. Pile egg whites on top of chocolate pie and using a spoon form some peaks. Make sure to get the egg whites completely to the edge of the crust... they call this sealing the edge.
12. Bake for approximately 20 minutes or until the meringue is golden brown.

JōZ Tip: WATCH VIDEO... this really helps with this recipe.

Buttermilk Pie
(Lemon or Maple flavor)

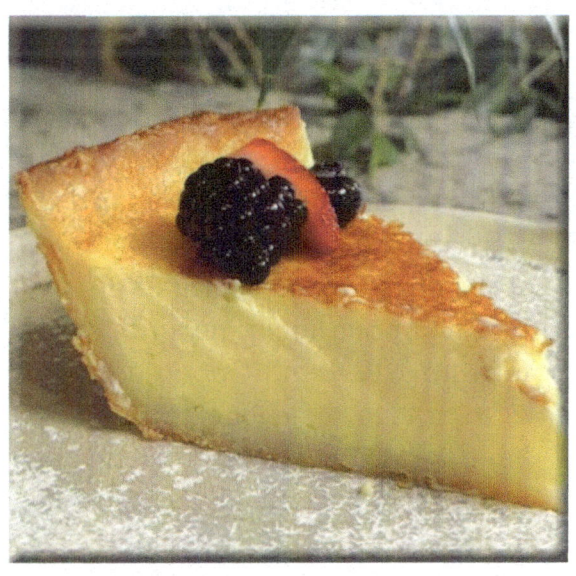

INGREDIENTS

1 JōZ pie crust uncooked (Recipe in cookbook)
8 Tbsp butter softened
300 g sugar
2 Tbsp GF flour*
2 Tbsp corn starch
¼ tsp salt
1 tsp vanilla
3 eggs
240 ml buttermilk
30 g of maple syrup or 2 tsp maple extract
ALT: lemon zest with a ½ tsp of lemon extract

1. Preheat oven to 350°F.
2. Prepare JōZ Pie Crust as directed and place in a 9-inch pie dish. Place in refrigerator.
3. In a large mixing bowl, on medium-high speed, beat butter and sugar until creamy. Turn speed to low, and add eggs one at a time until combined and mixture is smooth and creamy.
4. In medium size bowl, whisk flour, salt, and cornstarch until combined.
5. Add flour mixture into butter/sugar mixture and beat on low until smooth.
6. Slowly pour in buttermilk and continue to mix until the filling is completely combined and smooth.
7. Add vanilla and either your maple or lemon selection. Continue to mix on LOW speed, until nice and creamy.
8. Remove pie crust from refrigerator and pour the filling into crust.
9. Cook for around 50 minutes. Let cool completely and refrigerate for at least 2 hours. Enjoy!

JōZ Tip: I use Cup 4 Cup™ for my flour. **DO NOT OVERCOOK!**

JōZ Cookie

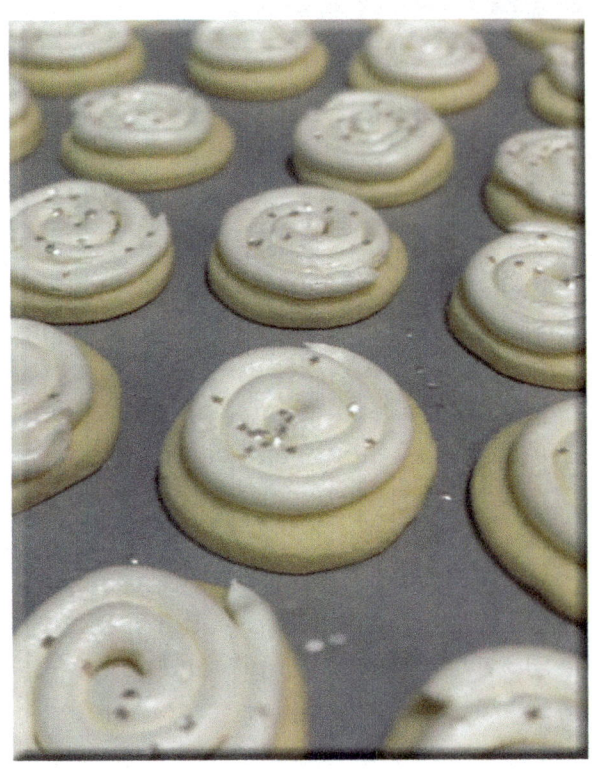

INGREDIENTS

- 300 g GF flour*
- 125 g sugar
- 1 tsp baking powder
- ½ tsp salt
- 42 g powdered sugar
- 6 Tbsp butter (salted)
- 4 oz cream cheese
- ½ tsp vanilla extract
- ½ tsp almond extract
- 1 extra large egg
- 1 Tbsp heavy cream

1. Preheat oven to 350°F.
2. In a large mixing bowl, whisk flour, sugar, baking powder, salt, and powdered sugar.
3. In a separate mixing bowl, add melted butter, softened cream cheese, extracts, egg, and heavy cream. Mix well with a hand mixer.
4. Make a well in the center of dry mixture and pour liquid mixture into dry mixture. Stir with a spoon until mixture starts to come together. Take your hand to finish mixing ingredients until the mixture becomes a ball of dough.
5. Refrigerate for about 10 minutes.
6. Take dough and put between parchment paper and roll out to about 1/4- 1/3 inch thick. Use a cookie cutter of your choice and place cookie onto a cookie sheet lined with parchment paper.
7. Bake for 10-12 minutes. Allow to cool before frosting.

JōZ Tip: I use Better Batter™ flour. Roll dough to your desired thickness.

JōZ Chocolate Cookie

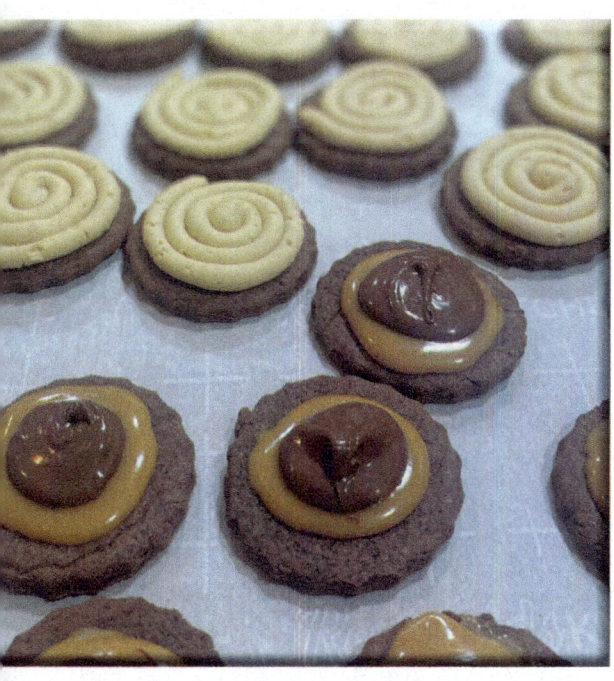

INGREDIENTS

260 g GF flour*
100 g sugar
1 3.4 oz box instant chocolate pudding
1 Tbsp extra dark cocoa
1 tsp baking powder
½ tsp salt
44 g powdered sugar
6 Tbsp butter (salted)
4 oz cream cheese
½ tsp vanilla extract
1 extra large egg
1 ½ Tbsp heavy cream

1. Preheat oven to 350°F.
2. In a large mixing bowl, whisk together flour, sugar, pudding, cocoa, baking powder, salt, and powdered sugar.
3. In a separate mixing bowl, add melted butter, softened cream cheese, extract, egg, and heavy cream. Mix well with a hand mixer.
4. Make a well in the center of dry mixture and pour liquid mixture into dry mixture. Stir with spoon until mixture starts to come together. Take your hand to finish mixing ingredients until the mixture becomes a ball of dough.
5. Refrigerate for about 10 minutes.
6. Take dough and put between parchment paper and roll out to about 1/4-1/3 inch thick. Use a cookie cutter of your choice and place cookie onto a cookie sheet lined with parchment paper.
7. Bake for 10-12 minutes. Allow to cool before frosting.

JōZ Tip: I use Better Batter™ flour. Roll dough to your desired thickness.

Chocolate Chip Cookies

INGREDIENTS

280 g GF flour*
1 tsp baking soda
1 tsp salt
48 g vanilla instance pudding mix
12 Tbsp butter (melted)
2 oz cream cheese (room temp)
85 g light brown sugar
85 g dark brown sugar
100 g sugar
½ tsp vanilla
2 egg
12 oz of chocolate chips
Nuts or additional different flavored chips (optional)

1. Using a large mixing bowl whisk flour, soda, and salt until combined. Set aside.
2. In a large stand mixing bowl, using a paddle attachment, mix on medium high butter, cream cheese, sugars, eggs, vanilla and pudding mix until combined.
3. Pour flour mixture into butter mixture and beat on **LOW** until mostly combined. Add in chips and nuts and continue to stir until dough is formed and all ingredients are well combined.
4. Line cookie sheet with parchment paper. Roll dough into balls and place on cookie sheet.
5. Place cookie sheet in the refrigerator for at least 15 minutes to chill.
5. Preheat oven to 375°F.
6. Remove cookies from the refrigerator and place them in oven and cook for 10-13 minutes depending on how soft or crispy you like your cookies.

JōZ Tip: I like to use King Arthur's™ Gluten Free flour. Chilling dough before cooking is super important.

For the Love of Gluten Free

Key Lime Cupcakes

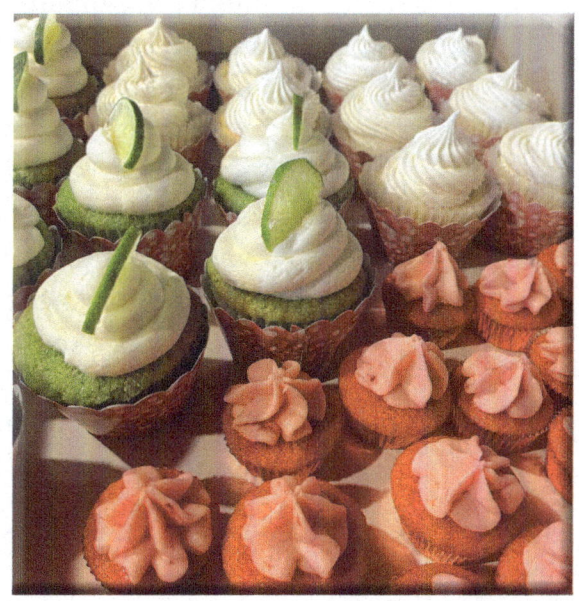

INGREDIENTS

CAKE INGREDIENTS

    285 g GF Flour*
    265 g sugar
    1 3 oz box Lime Jello
    1 tsp baking powder
    1 tsp soda
    ½ tsp salt
    160 ml orange juice (room temp)
    224 ml canola oil
    4 eggs (room temp)
    zest and juice from 4-5 key limes
    120 g of sour cream (room temp)
    3 drops of lime oil*
    green food coloring (optional)

LIME CREAM CHEESE FROSTING INGREDIENTS

    2 sticks of unsalted butter (softened)
    8 oz block of cream cheese (softened)
    4-6 cups of powdered sugar
    2-4 Tbsp heavy whipping cream
    1/2 tsp vanilla
    Juice from 2-3 key limes

CUPCAKES

1. Preheat oven to 350°F.
2. Line your cupcake pan with liners, making sure to leave a few open cups (see video).

For the Love of Gluten Free

3. Using a large mixing bowl, sift together flour, sugar, Jello, baking powder, soda and salt. Set aside.
4. In a separate mixing bowl, whisk together orange juice, canola oil, eggs, zest and juice from limes.
5. Pour liquid mixture into dry mixture and stir with a large spoon until smooth.
6. Add sour cream and continue to stir until combined.
7. Add lime oil and food coloring and stir until all ingredients are combined and batter is smooth.
8. Fill the cupcake liners 2/3 full. Do not overfill.
9. Fill the empty spots with water.
10. Bake for 15-17 minutes until a toothpick is inserted and comes out clean.
11. Let cool completely before frosting.

FROSTING

1. Using a stand mixer, whip butter on high for 5 minutes.
2. Add 2 oz of cream cheese at a time until well combined. Beat on high for 2-3 minutes.
3. Add powdered sugar slowly into mixer alternating with heavy cream. Add vanilla and lime juice and beat until desired thickness.
4. Frost cupcakes.

JōZ Tip: I recommend Bob's Red Mill™ Gluten Free flour. I used lime oil from Young Living™. The video for this recipe is very helpful.

Strawberry Cupcakes

INGREDIENTS

280 g GF Flour*
300 g sugar
1 3oz box Strawberry Jello
1 tsp baking powder
1 tsp soda
½ tsp salt
185 ml orange juice (room temp)
224 ml canola oil
4 eggs (room temp)
120 g sour cream (room temp)
1 tsp strawberry emulsion or extract
1 tsp vanilla extract

CAKE

1. Preheat oven to 350°F.
2. Line your cupcake pan with liners, making sure to leave a few open cups (see video).
3. Using a large mixing bowl, sift together flour, sugar, Jello, baking powder, soda and salt. Set aside.
4. In a separate mixing bowl, whisk together orange juice, canola oil, and eggs.
5. Pour liquid mixture into dry mixture and stir with a large spoon until smooth.
6. Add sour cream and continue to stir until combined.
7. Add emulsion and vanilla and continue to stir until all ingredients are combined and batter is smooth.
8. Fill the cupcake liners 2/3 full. Do not overfill.
9. Fill the empty spots with water.
10. Bake for 15-17 minutes until a toothpick is inserted and comes out clean.
11. Let cool completely before frosting.

FROSTING

1. Using a stand mixer, whip butter on high for 5 minutes.
2. Add 2oz of cream cheese at a time until well combined. Beat on high for 2-3 minutes.
3. Add powdered sugar slowly into mixer, alternating with heavy cream. Add vanilla and beat until desired thickness.
4. Frost cupcakes

JōZ Tip: I recommend Bob's Red Mill™ Gluten Free flour. I use strawberry emulsion. The video for this recipe is very helpful.

Pumpkin Cupcakes or Muffins

INGREDIENTS

- 290 g GF Flour*
- 1 Tbsp baking powder
- 1 tsp salt
- 200 g sugar
- 100 g dark brown sugar
- 3 eggs
- 4 Tbsp butter (melted)
- 200 ml canola oil
- 244 g canned pumpkin
- 120 g sour cream
- 1 tsp cinnamon

1. Preheat oven to 350°F.
2. Line your cupcake pan with liners, making sure to leave a few open cups (see video).
3. Using a large mixing bowl, whisk together flour, baking powder, and salt. Set aside.
4. In a separate mixing bowl, using a hand mixer, mix together melted butter and oil. Add eggs and beat until creamy. Add sugar, brown sugar, and canned pumpkin and beat until smooth and creamy.
5. Pour liquid mixture into dry mixture and stir with a large spoon until smooth.
6. Add sour cream and continue to stir until combined.
7. Add cinnamon and continue to stir until all ingredients are combined and batter is smooth.
8. Fill the cupcake liners 2/3 full. **DO NOT OVERFILL!**
9. Fill the empty spots with water.
10. Bake for 15-17 minutes until a toothpick is inserted and comes out clean.
11. Let cool.

JōZ Tip: I recommend Bob's Red Mill™ Gluten Free flour. I will frost these with cream cheese frosting if I want a cupcake or I will top with a brown sugar crumble if I want to serve muffins.

Mini Cheesecake & Fried Cheesecake Bites

MINI CHEESECAKES

1 JōZ GF Graham Cracker Crust recipe (Recipe in cookbook)
16 oz cream cheese (softened)
120 g sugar
2 eggs (room temp)
120 g sour cream (room temp)
pinch of salt
1 tsp vanilla paste

FRIED CHEESECAKE BITES

186 g GF Flour*
50 g sugar
1 tsp baking powder
240 ml milk (room temp)
5 oz club soda
Canola oil for frying

MINI CHEESECAKES

1. Preheat oven to 350°F.
2. Prepare JōZ Graham Cracker Crust per recipe. Set aside.
3. Line your cupcake pans with liners, making sure you leave a few open (see video).
4. Using a spoon, add approximately a tablespoon of graham cracker crust mixture to each liner and press with spoon to bottom of liner. Set aside.
5. In a large mixing bowl, beat cream cheese with mixer until smooth. Add sugar, salt and sour cream and continue to beat with mixer.
6. Turn mixer to low and add one egg at a time until combined.
7. Add vanilla and whip for a few more seconds on low.
8. Fill cupcake liners 2/3 full. Do not overfill. I like to leave a few open holes and fill with water.
9. Cook for approximately 16-18 minutes until cheesecakes are set. DO NOT OVERCOOK.

JōZ Tip: I like to refrigerate for a few hours. However, some people like to eat them warm. Top with your favorite topping. Enjoy! Video offers some great tips.

Fried Cheesecake Bites

1. Cut mini cheesecakes into fourths. Place back into the refrigerator and make sure they are very cold.
2. In a large mixing bowl, whisk together flour, sugar, and baking powder. Slowly stir in milk until combined and smooth. Place in the refrigerator to chill. (At least 30 minutes)
3. When ready to prepare, heat oil to 360-370°. Take your batter out of refrigerator and add in club soda until batter is thin enough to dip bites. Using a fork, dip bites into batter and then into oil. Let cook until golden brown. Approximately 1-2 minutes. Turn and allow to cook another 1-2 minutes.
4. Remove from oil and place on a wire wrack or paper towel lined plate. Allow to cool. Serve with your favorite dipping sauce.

JōZ Tip: I use Cup 4 Cup™ or King Arthur™ Gluten Free Flour

Blueberry Lime Bread

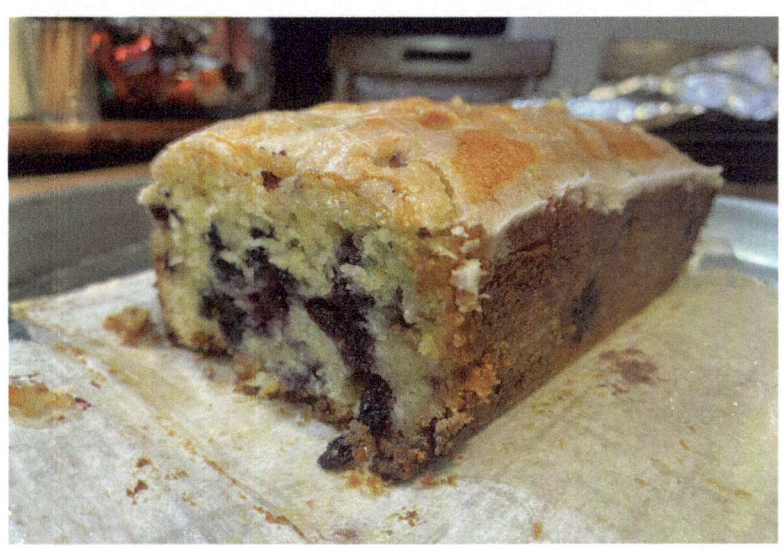

INGREDIENTS

280 g GF Flour
250 g sugar
1 Tbsp GF flour to coat blueberries
1 Tbsp sugar to coat blueberries
1 tsp baking powder
½ tsp salt
200 g fresh blueberries (rinsed)
160 ml milk (room temp)
140 ml canola oil
2 eggs (room temp)
Zest from 1 lime
Juice from lime divided
3 drops lime oil*

LIME GLAZE

3 Tbsp butter
Approximately 3-4 large spoonful of powdered sugar
3 Tbsp water
Juice from ½ of lime

ALTERNATE GLAZE

Lime Cream Cheese Frosting
2 sticks of unsalted butter (softened)
8 oz block of cream cheese (softened)
4-6 cups of powdered sugar
2-4 Tbsp heavy whipping cream
1 tsp vanilla
Juice from 2-3 key limes

For the Love of Gluten Free

1. Preheat oven to 350°F.
2. Line two, 8x4 loaf pans with parchment paper and lightly spray corners. Set aside.
3. In a small zippy bag, coat rinsed blueberries with 1 Tbsp sugar and 1 Tbsp flour and set aside.
4. In a large mixing bowl, whisk together flour, sugar, baking powder, and salt.
5. In a medium bowl, mix milk, oil, eggs, and zest.
6. Pour liquid mixture into dry mixture and stir will large spoon until combined.
7. Sift all flour and sugar off blueberries before folding blueberries into batter.
8. Gently stir in juice from ½ of lime and lime oil.
9. Using your scale, pour equal amounts into your 8x4 loaf pans.
10. Before placing bread in oven, place a few blueberries on top. Bake for 50-60 minutes.
11. While bread is baking, mix up Lime Glaze or Lime Cream Cheese frosting.

JōZ Tip: I use Bob's Red Mill™ Gluten Free Baking Flour

Banana Chocolate Chip Bread

INGREDIENTS

4 Tbsp melted salted butter
70 ml milk (room temp)
2 eggs (room temp)
4 extra ripe bananas
150 g of sugar
48 g of brown sugar
280 g of GF flour*
1 tsp baking powder
½ tsp baking soda
½ tsp salt
1 tsp cinnamon
1 tsp vanilla or vanilla paste
200 g of chocolate chips coated in GF flour (optional)

1. Preheat oven to 350°F.
2. Line two loaf pans with parchment paper and spray lightly in corners with nonstick spray.
3. In a large mixing bowl, whisk together flour, baking powder, salt, and baking soda.
4. In a medium mixing bowl, using a hand mixer, combine melted butter, milk, eggs, bananas, and sugars until smooth.
5. Pour wet ingredients into dry ingredients and using a large spoon, stir until smooth.
6. Add cinnamon and vanilla and stir until combined.
7. Fold in chocolate chips making sure to sift off the flour before you add them.
8. Using your scale, pour equal amounts into loaf pans.
9. Before placing bread in oven, place a few chocolate chips on top. Bake for 50-60 minutes.

JōZ Tip: I use Bob's Red Mill™ Gluten Free Baking Flour.

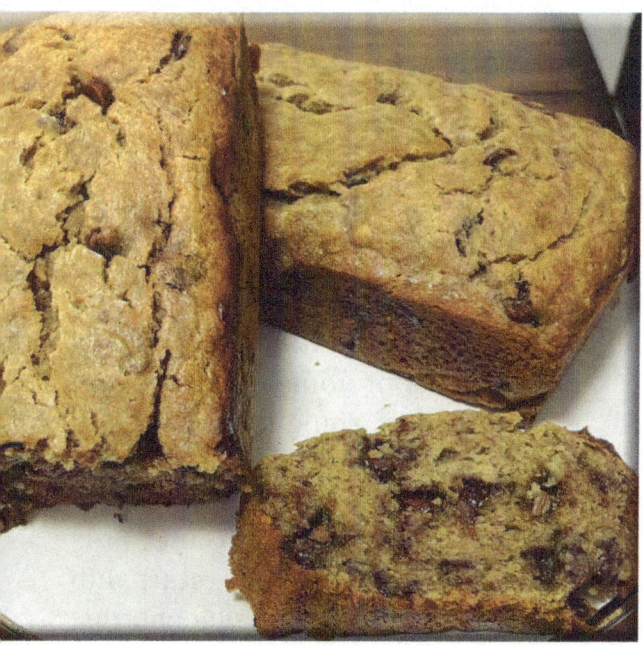

JōZ Churro's

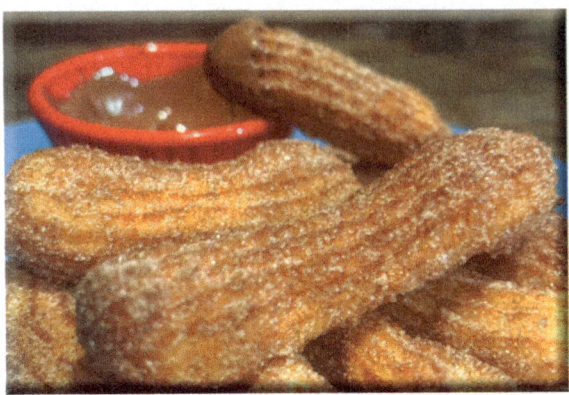

INGREDIENTS

240 ml water
6 Tbsp unsalted butter
2 Tbsp sugar
½ tsp salt
140 g gluten free flour*
15 g cornstarch
3 eggs (room temperature)
Canola Oil for frying
½ tsp vanilla paste

INGREDIENTS FOR CHURRO COATING

100 g white sugar
2 tsp cinnamon

1. In a small mixing bowl, whisk flour and cornstarch together and set aside.
2. Using a medium saucepan, add water, butter, sugar, and salt and bring to a low boil on medium high heat.
3. Turn heat down to low and add flour mixture and with large spoon/spatula stir until dough forms into a ball. This takes about 2-3 minutes.
4. Remove from heat and let cool for about 5-10 minutes.
5. Using a handheld mixture, add 1 egg at a time and beat on medium low speed until incorporated. Repeat this step until all eggs have been added. Add vanilla paste.
6. Continue to beat at medium speed until the dough becomes smooth.
7. Transfer dough to a pastry bag fitted with a large open star tip and set aside.
8. Using a large skillet, heat oil to 360° F.
9. While oil is heating, mix sugar and cinnamon in a dish large enough to toss churros.
10. When oil reaches the desired temperature, carefully pipe out about 4-5 inches of dough and fry for about 4 minutes turning every minute or so.
11. When they are golden brown, remove and place on a paper towel to remove excess oil and then coat in the cinnamon sugar mixture.
12. Serve warm with Nutella, warm caramel sauce, or your favorite sweet dipping sauce. You can also fill with cream or pudding.

JōZ Tip: I Use Cup 4 Cup™ Gluten Free flour. If this is your first time, start with small batches as well as smaller churros. Also, video is super helpful!

MAIN COURSES

Beef Tips and Mashed Potatoes

INGREDIENTS

- 2 lbs of beef stew meat
- 2 Tbsp of canola oil
- 2 Tbsp butter
- 1/2 onion chopped
- 1 clove chopped garlic
- 360 ml water
- 120 ml beef broth
- 3 Tbsp GF soy sauce*
- 4 Tbsp Worcestershire sauce*
- 1/2 tsp salt
- 1 tsp black pepper

BEEF TIPS

1. In a large skillet on medium heat, add oil, butter, sautéed onions, and garlic for a couple of minutes.
2. Turn up the heat and add your stew meat and brown on both sides. This takes just a few minutes.
3. Add water, broth, soy sauce, Worcestershire sauce, salt, and pepper, and bring to a low simmer.
4. Stir slightly, cover and turn heat down to low.
5. Cook on low heat for 1 ½ -2 hours until meet is tender.

JōZ Tip: The biggest mistake made is not cooking the beef long enough. The meat should fall apart.

Brown Gravy

INGREDIENTS

- 1 Tbsp butter
- 1 clove of garlic
- 2 cups of beef broth
- ½ tsp onion powder
- 1 tsp salt
- 2 tsp Worcestershire Sauce
- 2-3 drops Kitchen Bouquet™ browning and seasoning sauce
- 4 Tbsp water
- 3 Tbsp corn starch

1. Using a medium saucepan, melt butter and sauté minced garlic for 1-2 mins.
2. Add broth, onion powder, salt, and Worcestershire sauce and bring to a simmer.
3. In a small bowl, mix water and corn starch then pour into saucepan and continue to whisk while sauce thickens.
4. Add a few drops of browning seasoning and simmer for 10 mins. Gravy is ready to serve.

JōZ Tip: If sauce becomes too thick add more broth to desired consistency.

Mashed Potatoes

- 5 large potatoes, peeled and cut into cubes
- Water
- 1 Tbsp salt
- 1 cloves fresh garlic minced
- 12 Tbsp stick butter
- 120 ml heavy cream
- Salt and Pepper

1. Peel and wash potatoes.
2. Cut into 1-inch cubes and add large boiler and cover potatoes with water and salt.
3. Cook on medium heat until potatoes have softened. If a fork goes in easily, they are ready.
4. In a small saucepan, over medium heat, melt butter and sauté garlic for a few minutes. Add heavy cream and heat on low until the mixture is nice and warm.
5. Drain water off potatoes and slowly add your warm cream a little at a time.
6. Add salt and pepper to taste.

JōZ Tip: Remember salt is your friend. Haha!

Baked Chicken and Shrimp Alfredo

ALFREDO INGREDIENTS

12 Tbsp of butter (salted)
3 cloves fresh garlic minced
3 c of heavy cream (room temp)
6 oz cream cheese (room temp and cut into small squares)
5 oz fresh shredded Parmesan cheese, (divided...set aside about 1 oz to sprinkle on top)
5 oz fresh shredded Mozzarella cheese, (divided...set aside about 1 oz to sprinkle on top)
Salt and Pepper to taste

CHICKEN AND SHRIMP

1 lb chicken tenderloins
1 12 oz pkg medium shrimp (raw, deveined and tail off)
4 Tbsp Butter (**divided**)
2 cloves of fresh minced garlic (**divided**)

PENNE PASTA (GLUTEN FREE)

12 oz GF Penne noodles
1 Tbsp salt
1 Tbsp olive oil

1. Preheat oven to 375°F.
2. Using kitchen shears or a knife, cut up chicken into bite size pieces.
3. In a large skillet, melt 2 Tbsp of butter and 1 tsp fresh minced garlic on medium heat. Add chicken and cook until the chicken is mostly done. Transfer chicken to a bowl.
4. Using the same skillet, melt 2 Tbsp of butter and 1 tsp fresh minced garlic on medium high heat. Add shrimp and cook until shrimp turns pink. This does not take long. Transfer to the bowl with chicken.
5. In a large boiler, bring water and salt to a low boil. Add noodles and oil and cook until pasta is cooked through but still has a slight resistance when you bite into it (al dente). Stir occasionally to prevent sticking. This takes about 10 minutes.
6. While pasta is cooking, take an extra-large skillet, melt 12 Tbsp of butter and 3 cloves of minced garlic on medium low heat.
7. Add heavy cream and bring to a low simmer. Make sure you keep heat low from this point on.

8. Add cream cheese and continue to cook on low. I use a rubber spatula to stir making sure it is not sticking to the bottom of the skillet.
9. Add 4 oz of Parmesan and 4 oz of Mozzarella and salt and pepper. Cook **slowly** until melted and your alfredo sauce is nice and creamy.
10. Drain water off pasta and transfer pasta to a 9x13 deep casserole dish.
11. Add Chicken and shrimp to top of pasta and poor alfredo sauce over top of ingredients. Take your spatula and gently fold mixture. Sprinkle Parmesan and Mozzarella on top and cover with foil.
12. Place it in oven and cook for approximately 15-20 minutes.

JōZ Tip: Serve with salad and some yummy GF garlic bread. Video is super helpful!

Grilled Chicken Fettuccine

ALFREDO INGREDIENTS

12 Tbsp butter (salted)
3 cloves fresh garlic minced
3 c of heavy cream (room temp)
6 oz cream cheese (room temp and cut into small squares)
4 oz fresh shredded Parmesan cheese
4 oz fresh shredded Mozzarella cheese
Salt and Pepper to taste

CHICKEN INGREDIENTS

Chicken breast or Chicken tenderloins
2 Tbsp melted butter
1 Tbsp olive oil
120 g Greek yogurt
1 Tbsp honey
1 pkg Italian seasoning
juice from ½ of lemon

FETTUCCINE PASTA (GLUTEN FREE)

12 oz GF Fettuccine noodles
1 Tbsp salt
1 Tbsp olive oil

1. Take chicken tenderloins and place them in a large zippy bag. (If using chicken breast, cut into strips).
2. In a small mixing bowl, whisk together butter, oil, honey, seasoning and lemon juice. Pour into zippy bag over chicken and marinate for at least an hour.
3. Heat grill to 375°F.
4. In a large boiler, bring water and salt to a low boil. Add noodles and oil and cook until pasta is cooked through but still has a slight resistance when you bite into it (al dente). Stir occasionally to prevent sticking. This takes about 14 minutes.
5. While pasta is cooking, take an extra-large skillet, melt 12 Tbsp of butter and 3 cloves of minced garlic on medium low heat.
6. Add heavy cream and bring to a low simmer. Make sure you keep heat low from this point on.
7. Add cream cheese and continue to cook on low. I use a rubber spatula to stir making sure it is not sticking to the bottom of the skillet.
8. Add 4 oz of Parmesan and 4 oz of Mozzarella and salt and pepper. Cook **slowly** until melted and your alfredo sauce is nice and creamy.

9. Place chicken on grill and cook approximately 8+ minutes, turning over after 4 minutes. Ensure the internal temperature of the chicken reaches 165°F.
10. When chicken is done, drain water off noodles.
11. Place noodles on plate and cover with alfredo sauce and top with grilled chicken.

JōZ Tip: Serve with salad and some yummy GF garlic bread. Video is helpful! Plus, you get to meet my sexy husband!

Chicken and Rice

INGREDIENTS

200 g (dry) rice
480 ml water
1 Tbsp salted butter
1 18 oz can of Mushroom soup*
120 ml milk
60 ml chicken broth
120 g sour cream
6 oz fresh shredded mozzarella cheese
Approximately 3 cups of fully cooked shredded chicken*
1 tsp salt
½ tsp pepper
Velvetta cheese

1. Using a large boiler, add rice, water, and butter and bring to a low boil. Turn the temperature down to low and cover with lid. Cook for 20-25 mins.
2. Remove from heat and add soup, milk, broth, sour cream, mozzarella cheese, chicken, salt, and pepper. Gently stir until everything is well combined.
3. Preheat oven to 350°F.
4. Pour mixture into a 9x13 dish and place it in oven. Bake for 15-20 minutes. Remove and add Velvetta cheese and place back in oven for 5 minutes. It is ready to serve.

JōZ Tip: I recommend boiling a whole chicken and using it in this dish. See video!

Gluten Free Pizza

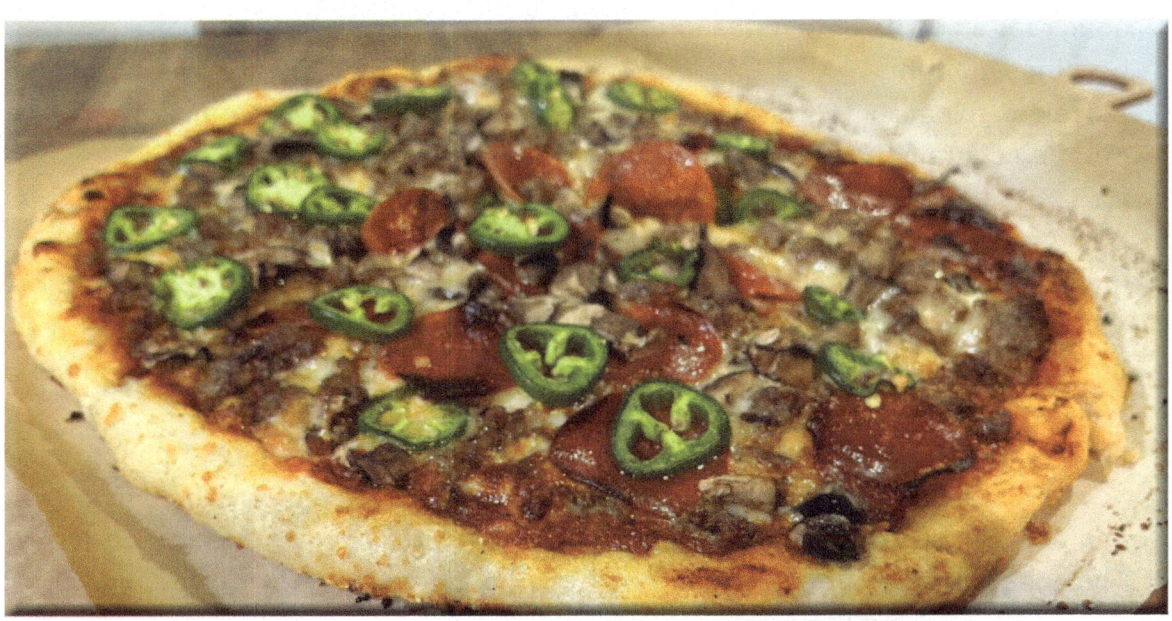

INGREDIENTS

- 180 g GF flour* Plus extra for rolling out dough
- 2 tsp salt
- 240 ml warm water (About 110° F.)
- 1 packet of dry active yeast (this is about 7 g or 2 tsp)
- 1 tsp sugar
- 1 tsp olive oil
- Your favorite pizza sauce
- 4 Tbsp butter (melted)
- Fresh garlic (minced)
- Mozzarella string cheese (optional)
- Fresh Mozzarella cheese (grated)
- Fresh Parmesan cheese (grated)
- 16 oz Italian sausage
- 8 oz pork sausage
- Pepperoni (as many as you like)
- Veggies, pineapple, and peppers (optional)

1. Using a medium bowl, stir warm water (make sure it's at least 105°-110°F), yeast and sugar. Set aside to activate.
2. Add flour and salt to a large stand mixing bowl.
3. When yeast is activated, add olive oil then pour into flour and turn on low, scraping down sides a few times until ingredients are combined. Turn speed to medium-high and mix for 6-8 minutes.

For the Love of Gluten Free

4. Liberally sprinkle flour on to counter. Spray rubber spatula with olive oil and scrape dough onto counter. Knead dough for a couple of minutes until it becomes smooth.
5. Place dough back into a large bowl or proofing container and cover. Let rise for 1 ½- 2 hours.
6. Using a large skillet cook sausage, drain off grease and set aside.
7. Place pizza stone in oven and preheat to 550° F.
8. When dough has risen to about double in size, sprinkle a small amount of flour or cornmeal on parchment paper and begin to roll dough into a circle. Thickness is up to you. I like a thin crust, so I roll it out thin.
9. Take Mozzarella string cheese and pull apart into quarters. Place around edge of pizza crust and roll dough over cheese creating a stuffed crust. This is optional.
10. In small boiler, melt butter and fresh minced garlic till warm. Spread liberally on top of pizza crust with pastry brush
11. Sprinkle some fresh grated parmesan cheese on top. (as much or as little as you want)
12. Place crust in oven for 3-4 minutes. Remove and add remaining toppings.
13. I start with my favorite pizza sauce. Followed by sausage, cheese, pepperonis, mushrooms, and jalapeños. But you do you!
14. Place back in oven for 15 minutes or until crust is nice and golden brown.
15. Remove and let stand for a few minutes.

JōZ Tip: I use Caputo™ Gluten Free flour. I get this on Amazon. **The video is a tremendous help**!

JōZ Chicken Tenders

INGREDIENTS

Chicken

1.5 lbs. of chicken tenderloins or chicken breast cut into strips (I even cut my tenderloins in smaller strips...they fry up better)
salt and pepper

Wet Ingredients

160 g Gluten Free Flour
2 Tbsp cornstarch
1 tsp salt
1 tsp baking powder
1 tsp garlic powder
½ tsp onion powder
½ tsp chili powder
½ tsp paprika
2 eggs
160 ml water
6-10 oz club soda (cold)

Dry Ingredients

300 g Gluten Free flour*
1 tsp salt
½ tsp garlic powder
½ tsp chili powder
½ tsp paprika
¼ tsp cayenne pepper
Oil for Frying

1. Lightly season chicken tenderloins/strips with salt and pepper and set aside.
2. Using a large mixing bowl whisk together flour, cornstarch, and seasonings. Add eggs and water and stir until combined. Stir in club soda until you reach a mildly thin batter. (about like cake batter)
3. Add chicken to the bowl and make sure every piece is coated in the batter. Cover and place bowl in refrigerator for at least an hour! (longer if possible)
4. Using a large pan, mix all your dry ingredients and set aside.
5. When ready to prepare, heat oil in a large skillet on medium high heat to 360-375° F.
6. Take chicken tenders and toss in flour mixture then carefully add to oil.
7. Cook chicken tenders for 2-3 minutes on each side. Make sure the internal temperature is at least 165°F.
8. Remove from oil and place on paper towel or wire rack to cool.

JōZ Tip: I like King Arthur™ GF flour or Pamela's™ GF flour for this recipe. Video is helpful!

Baked Fish

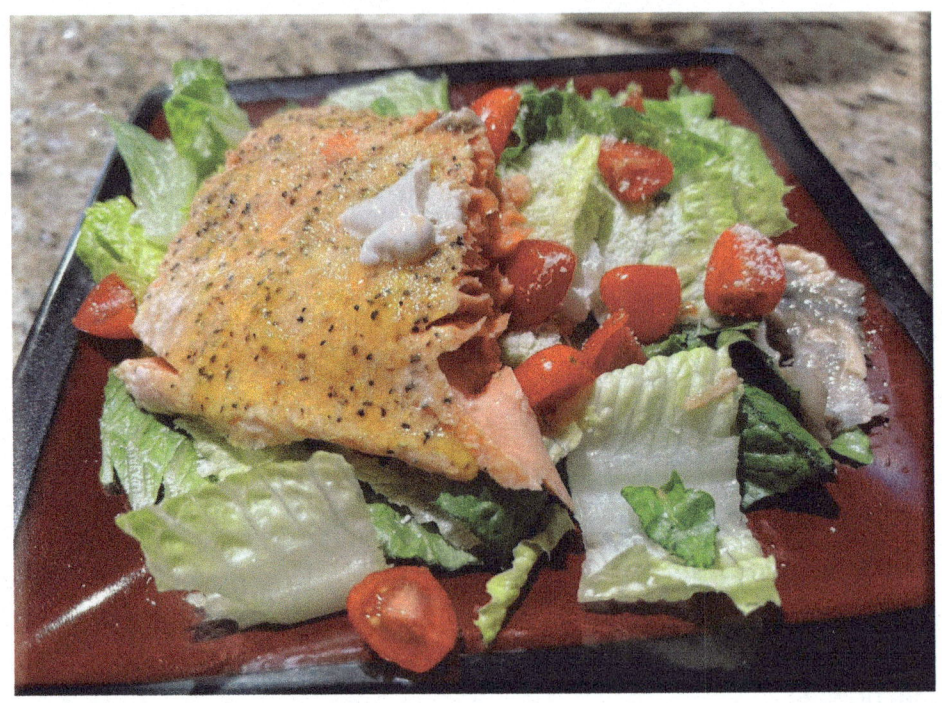

INGREDIENTS

1 whole salmon or trout or 4-6 individual pieces of fish
1 stick of salted butter melted
1 lemon sliced
lemon pepper seasoning
Slap Yo Mama™ seasoning or seasoning of your choice

1. Heat oven to 400°F.
2. Line large sheet pan with foil. Place fish skin down and pour melted butter over top of fish.
3. Sprinkle liberally with seasoning with as many different seasonings as you wish. Place sliced lemon on top of fish.
4. Cover with foil and cook for 20-25 minutes depending on the size of fish. **DO NOT OVERCOOK!**

JōZ Tip: Video has some great information and tips.

For the Love of Gluten Free

Fried Fish

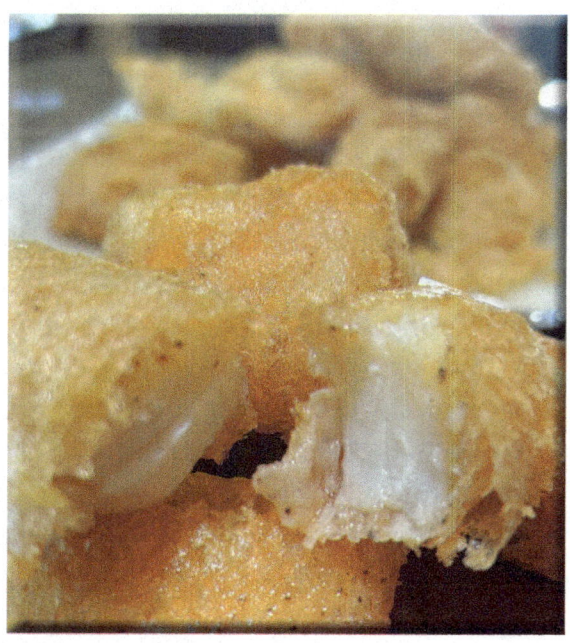

INGREDIENTS

1.5 lbs of white fish (I like cod, tilapia, and haddock)
124 g GF Flour* plus extra for dredging
40 g super fine white rice flour
16 g cornstarch
½ tsp salt
2 tsp baking powder
2 tsp paprika
½ tsp onion powder
1 ½ tsp Slap Yo Mama™ seasoning
1 large egg (slightly beaten)
1 Tbsp oil
6-10 oz club soda (cold)
Oil for frying

1. Cut up fish into chunks. Place chunks in a large zip bag and coat with GF flour and salt/pepper.
2. In a large mixing bowl, mix all dry ingredients. Add egg, oil, and club soda and stir until batter is smooth. You want the batter to be thin and NOT thick.
3. In a large skillet, heat canola oil to approximately 360°. Take chunks of fish and dip in batter covering completely and add to heated oil. Fry for 2-3 minutes on each side OR if deep frying approximately 4 minutes.
4. Remove from the fryer and place on a rack or paper towel. Slightly salt and let cool for a minute or two and serve warm.

JōZ Tip: I like King Arthur™ GF flour or Pamela's™ GF flour for this recipe. For white rice flour I like Authentic Foods™ White Rice Flour Superfine or Bob's Red Mills™ White Rice Flour. If possible, try and find some fresh fish. Totally makes a difference.

Shrimp Tacos

INGREDIENTS

208 g mayonnaise
2 limes
2 tsp sugar
½ tsp garlic powder
½ tsp salt
¼ tsp pepper
dash of cayenne pepper
dash of chili powder
½ Tajin™ classic seasoning
1 cabbage chopped or shredded*
Fresh cilantro
1-2 jalapeños chopped
1 bag of small raw shrimp (thawed, deveined and tail off)
1 Tbsp JōZ Mexican seasoning (recipe in cookbook) or your favorite GF taco seasoning
Olive oil
2 Tbsp butter
JōZ corn tortillas (Recipe in cookbook) or your favorite brand of corn tortillas
Cotija grated cheese
Spicy mayo or siracha (Optional)

1. Place shrimp in bowl and drizzle with olive oil. Coat shrimp with taco seasoning. Set aside.
2. Using a medium mixing bowl, mix mayo, sugar, and all seasonings. Add the juice of 1 lime and stir until nice and smooth. Set aside.
3. In a separate bowl, mix chopped cabbage, fresh cilantro, and chopped jalapeño. Set aside.
4. Make **JōZ** corn tortillas per recipe. Place in a tortilla holder to keep warm.
5. Using a large skillet, melt butter on medium high heat. Add shrimp to skillet and cook for 3-4 minutes. **DO NOT OVERCOOK!** Remove from heat and cover to keep warm.
6. Take your liquid ingredients and drizzle over cabbage mixture. I like to do this right before I'm ready to assemble my tacos.
7. Taking a corn tortilla, add your shrimp and cabbage mixture and top with Cotija cheese and spicy mayo or siracha if desired.

JōZ Tip: Using homemade corn tortillas makes a world of difference. Don't add too much liquid to your cabbage…it will make it soggy. You want it to remain crisp. Also, I just buy the 12 oz bag of cabbage to make it simpler. Serve with JōZ Spanish rice and refried beans.

JōZ's Chaunklas

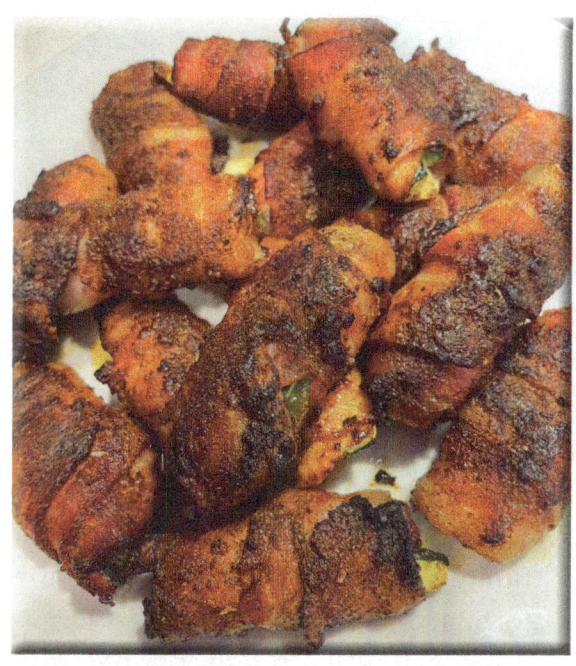

INGREDIENTS

1 Beef filet steak
1 Chicken breast
2 Jalapenos (rinsed and deseeded)
1 Zucchini (rinsed)
1 Pkg of Bacon (slices cut in half)
JōZ Mexican Seasoning or your favorite GF taco seasoning
1 Tbsp brown sugar

1. Preheat oven to 425°F
2. Cut steak and chicken into strips about 3 inches long. Season lightly with taco seasoning and set aside.
3. Cut jalapenos and zucchinis into strips about 3 inches long.
4. Line a cookie sheet with foil and spray with nonstick spray.
4. Take a piece of beef or chicken, jalapeno and zucchini and wrap with half a piece of bacon and place on cookie sheet. Repeat until all meat is gone. (may have a few veggies left)
5. Using a small bowl, take 2 Tbsp of Mexican seasoning and 1 Tbsp of brown sugar and mix with fork. Sprinkle over Chaunklas making sure to cover all sides.
6. Place in oven and cook for 15 minutes. Remove from the oven and turn Chaunklas over. Place back in oven and cook another 15-20 minutes.
7. Remove from oven and let cool slightly and serve with ranch dressing, sour cream or JōZ guacamole.

JōZ Tip: Thin cut bacon is recommended, as it wraps and cooks more efficiently than thicker cuts. Refer to the video for assembly instructions and additional tips. These can be served as appetizers or paired with Spanish rice and refried beans for a meal.

For the Love of Gluten Free

Deb and Seedie's Arizona Tacos

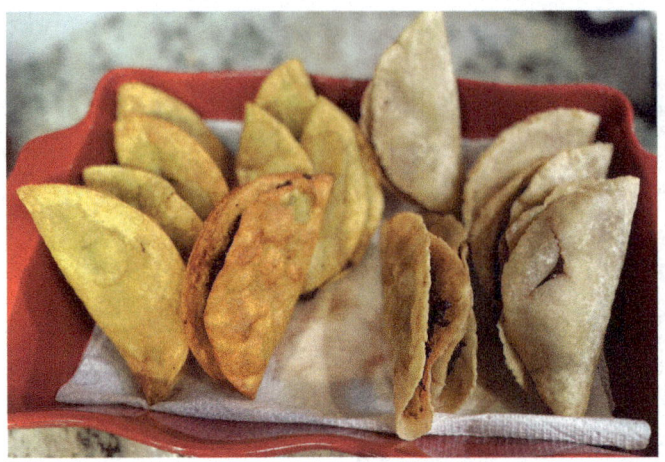

INGREDIENTS

1-1.5 lbs of good quality ground beef
1 dozen JōZ corn tortillas (recipe in cookbook) or your favorite brand of corn tortillas
salt, pepper, and garlic to taste
3 cups of chopped lettuce
2 cups shredded cheese (Colby Jack or Chedder)
1 cup of diced tomatoes
Salsa
Other optional toppings (cilantro, radishes, Cotija cheese, sour cream, jalapenos)

1. Using a large skillet, heat oil to 370°F.
2. While oil is heating, press ground beef firmly with your fingers onto 1/2 of the tortilla.
3. Season beef with salt, pepper, and garlic.
4. Gently place taco into grease, beef filled side last, folding gently as bottom side heats and softens. Cook 1-2 minutes.
5. Flip taco to beef filled side and cook additional 1-2 minutes until taco is golden brown.
6. Remove taco and allow to drain.
7. Fill with desired toppings and ENJOY!

 Deb & Seedie Tip: Do not place beef on tortillas and let sit for long before you fry. The tortillas will tend to get soggy.

To make these delicious tacos it is best to watch the video. You will love meeting Deb, one of my BFF's!

Pigs In A Blanket

INGREDIENTS

1 Serving of JōZ crescent rolls (Recipe in cookbook)
8 hotdogs or 24 mini cocktail wieners
melted butter
salt
mustard and ketchup for dipping

1. Prepare JōZ crescent roll dough as directed.
2. Preheat oven to 400°F
3. Line a baking sheet with parchment paper and spray lightly with nonstick spray.
4. Roll out crescent roll dough and cut into 8 large triangles or 24 min triangles.
5. Place wiener at the largest end of the triangle and roll towards the smallest.
6. Place on baking sheet and brush melted butter over dough with pastry brush. Sprinkle with a smidge of salt.
7. Bake for 20-25 minutes until golden brown. Mini's take less time.
8. Remove from oven and cool for 5-10 minutes and enjoy with your favorite dipping sauce.

JōZ Tip: Video is a great help. I have used JōZ puff pastry and JōZ pretzel dough in this recipe as well, and they are all great! You can also roll dough out into a "rope" and wrap it around the wieners.

Chicken Fried Steak Bites

INGREDIENTS

- 1 lb cubed steak tenderized
- 240-360 ml buttermilk
- 2 eggs
- Gluten Free flour used for dredging* (as much as you need)
- 1 tsp salt
- 1 tsp pepper
- 1 Tbsp Slap Yo Mama™ seasoning
- Canola oil for frying

1. Using kitchen shears or a sharp knife, cut cubed steak into bites size pieces and season with salt and pepper. Allow bites to come to room temperature.
2. In a large 9x13 dish, pour some flour, salt, pepper and Slap Yo Mama™ seasoning and whisk together. Set aside.
3. In a large bowl, whisk together buttermilk and eggs and allow them to come to room temperature as well.
5. Slightly toss steak bites in flour and then place them in buttermilk and allow to soak for at least 30 minutes.
6. When ready to prepare, take a large skillet and heat oil to 360-375° F.
7. When ready to fry, take bites and place them back in the flour mixture and make sure they are coated well.
8. Place bites in oil and fry for 3-4 minutes. This does not take long. **DO NOT OVERCOOK!**

JōZ Tip: I like to use King Arthur™ or Pamela's™ GF flour blend. If you are using a deep fryer, it only takes about 2-3 minutes. The video has a nice bonus recipe! Check it out!

For the Love of Gluten Free

Steak Bites

INGREDIENTS

1 Ribeye steak
2 Filet steaks
Edes™ Steak Seasoning or steak seasoning of your choice
3-4 sticks salted butter
2-3 cloves garlic chopped up

1. Cut up steaks into 2-inch size pieces and season with Edes™ seasoning or seasoning of your choice. Let sit at room temperature for a few hours if possible.
2. When ready to prepare steak, melt 3-4 sticks of butter with fresh garlic. Do not bring to a boil...just melt it.
3. Start heating your grill or griddle to high heat...at least 450° or hotter.
4. Take bites and soak them in butter for 3 minutes or so. Remove and immediately put on grill or griddle for approximately 4 mins flipping after about 2 mins. **PLEASE DO NOT OVERCOOK!** 😊
5. Remove from grill and enjoy with a baked potato, salad and some GF bread!

JōZ Tip: Try and get good quality beef. Video is super helpful, and you get to meet my sexy husband.

Spanish Rice

INGREDIENTS

60 ml Olive oil
400 g extra-long grain rice*
3-4 cloves of fresh garlic (minced)
32 oz chicken broth
100-120 g of Taco sauce*
1 tsp salt
½ tsp pepper
¼ tsp cummin

1. Using a large skillet (make sure to use one with a lid) heat oil on medium high heat.
2. Add rice and cook for approximately 2 minutes. The rice will be slightly browned.
3. Add minced garlic and cook another minute, stirring rice with a spatula.
4. Add broth, taco sauce, salt, pepper, and cummin. Stir slightly making sure everything is combined.
5. Reduce heat to low and cover with lid.
6. Cook for 20-25 minutes. (without peaking)
7. Remove the lid and toss rice gently making sure it is done. (Take a bite to make sure rice is soft and yummy) If it is still a little hard, place the lid back on and cook another 5-10 minutes.

JōZ Tip: Make sure you use a good quality rice. It does make a difference. I like to use Ortega Taco sauce™.

Onion Rings

INGREDIENTS

2 sweet onions (cut in slices)
GF flour✱ for dredging onions
180 g GF flour✱
60 g brown rice flour✱
1 tsp baking powder
½ tsp salt
½ tsp sugar
½ tsp paprika
200 ml milk (room temp)
56 ml canola oil
1 egg (room temp)
3-5 oz club soda✱ (cold)
Canola oil for frying
NOTE: If you are dairy free, replace the milk with more club soda

1. Cut onions into slices and place them in a large dish and sprinkle with some GF flour.
2. Using a medium size bowl, whisk together flour, brown rice flour, baking powder, salt, and sugar.
2. In a separate small bowl, mix milk, oil and egg until combined.
3. Pour liquid into dry ingredients and stir with spoon until combined. Place batter in refrigerator for at least 30 minutes.
4. Using a large skillet or deep fryer, heat oil to 360-375° F.
5. Remove batter from the refrigerator and add club soda, stirring until you reach a thin runny batter.
6. Take an onion, dip in batter, and carefully place into fryer.
7. Cook for 1-2 minutes before flipping over. Cook another 1-2 minutes until golden brown. If using a deep fryer, cook for 3-4 minutes or until golden brown.
8. Place on a cooling rack or sheet pan lined with a paper towel. Salt to your liking! ENJOY!

JōZ Tip: I like to use King Arthur™ or Pamela's™ GF flour blend and for the brown rice flour I like either Bob's Red Mill™ brown rice flour or Authentic Foods™ Brown Rice Flour Superfine. Also, you want your batter relatively thin. It thickens as you fry the onion rings. If you are dairy free, replace all milk with club soda.

For the Love of Gluten Free

Broccoli and Rice Casserole

INGREDIENTS

- 270 g of rice (rinsed)
- 600 ml water
- 1 tsp salt
- 3 Tbsp butter (divided)
- 1 18 oz Progresso™ Creamy Mushroom Soup
- 120 ml milk
- 120 ml heavy cream
- 16 oz broccoli cuts or chopped broccoli
- 16 oz of original Velveeta cheese
- Salt and Pepper

1. Preheat oven to 375°.
2. Using a large boiler, add rice, water, salt, and 1 Tbsp butter. Stir with a fork and bring to a boil. Turn heat down to simmer and cover. Cook for approximately 15-20 mins.
3. While rice is cooking, take a medium size saucepan, heat 2 Tbsp butter, soup, milk or cream and salt and pepper until warm. Add cheese and heat very slowly until melted, stirring occasionally.
4. Using a deep-dish casserole dish, spread cooked rice over bottom of dish, top with broccoli cuts or chopped broccoli. Pour cheesy soup mixture on top.
5. Using a spoon, gently stir until combined.
6. Cover with foil and place in oven to bake for approximately 15- 20 minutes.

JōZ Tip: Make sure you use filtered or bottled water to cook your rice in if you do not have well water.

I recommend using a good quality brand of long grained rice.

Santa Fe Soup

INGREDIENTS

1-2 lbs of hamburger meat
Green chiles (as many as you like)
½ small onion (chopped)
1 15 oz can pinto beans (rinsed and drained)
1 15 oz can fresh whole kernel corn (drained)
1 15oz can white hominy (drained)
1 10 oz can of RO-TEL™
1 14.5 oz can petite diced tomatoes
Beef broth (however much you desired)
16 oz Velvetta cheese

1. Using a large skillet, brown hamburger meat with green chiles and onions.
2. While meat is cooking, take a large pot and add beans, corn, hominy, RO-TEL™, and tomatoes. I like to add about 2 cups of broth at this point.
3. When the meat is done, drain grease and add to pot.
4. Cook on medium high heat for 10-15 mins. Turn heat down to low and let simmer for another 10 mins.
5. Cut up Velvetta into small chunks and add to the soup. Make sure the temperature is turned down to low. Soup is ready to serve when cheese is melted.

JoZ Tip: Make sure you rinse and drain the beans before cooking them. Also, if heat is too high when you add cheese, it could scorch and burn easily. If you don't want thick soup just add more broth.

Taco Soup

INGREDIENTS

- 1-2 lbs of ground beef (depends on how meaty you want it)
- 2 Tbsp JōZ Mexican seasoning or your favorite GF taco seasoning
- ½ diced onion (optional)
- 8 oz green chiles
- 1 packet of ranch dressing seasoning
- 1 15 oz can of fresh whole kernel corn (drained)
- 1 15 oz can of pinto beans (rinsed and drained)
- 1 15 oz can of black beans (rinsed and drained)
- 1 14.5 can of petite diced tomatoes
- 1 10 oz can of RO-TEL™
- 32 oz beef broth

1. Using a large skillet, brown hamburger meat, green chiles, and onions. Add about a cup of beef broth and taco seasoning and continue to cook until meat is done.
2. While the meat is cooking, take a large pot and add beans, corn, RO-TEL™, tomatoes, and ranch dip seasoning. I like to add beef broth at this point.
3. When the meat is done, add it to pot. Cook on medium high heat for 15 mins. Turn heat down to low and simmer for another 10 mins. Soup is ready to serve.

JōZ Tip: Make sure you rinse and drain beans. Also, I love to top with Pepper Jack cheese or Monterey Jack cheese. If you don't want a thick soup just add more broth.

BREADS, PASTRIES & CRUST

Corn Bread

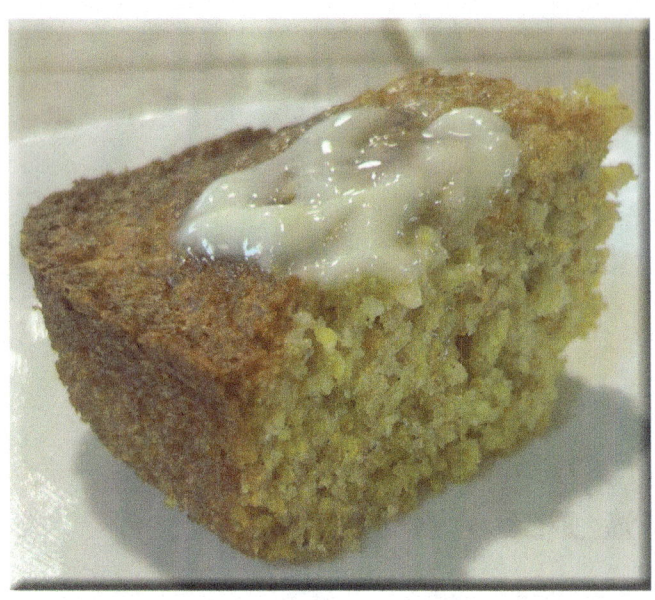

INGREDIENTS

- 152 g GF Cornmeal*
- 140 g GF flour*
- 66 g sugar
- 2 tsp baking powder
- ½ tsp baking soda
- ½ tsp salt
- 240 ml milk (room temp)
- 6 Tbsp butter melted (DIVIDED)
- 2 eggs (room temp)
- 1-2 Tbsp honey (optional)

1. Preheat oven to 375°.
2. Using a large mixing bowl, whisk together cornmeal, flour, sugar, baking powder, soda, and salt. Set aside.
3. In separate mixing bowl, mix milk and 4 Tbsp of melted butter until combined. Add eggs and continue to stir until combined.
4. Pour wet ingredients into dry ingredients. Using a large spoon, stir till ingredients are combined.
5. Add warmed honey if desired.
6. Add 2 Tbsp of butter to a 10-inch cast iron skillet and place it in the oven for five minutes to melt.
7. Remove cast iron skillet from the oven with melted butter and poor batter in immediately.
8. Place back in oven and cook until toothpick is inserted in the middle and comes out clean... Approximately 30 mins.

JōZ Tip: I've had success with both Cup 4 Cup™ Gluten Free flour and Bob's Red Mill™ Gluten Free Baking Flour. I use Bob's Red Mill™ Cornmeal medium grind for the cornmeal. If you don't like sweet cornbread, leave out the honey. Always use a cast iron skillet or metal pan. It does make a difference! Don't forget to watch the video!

Puff Pastry

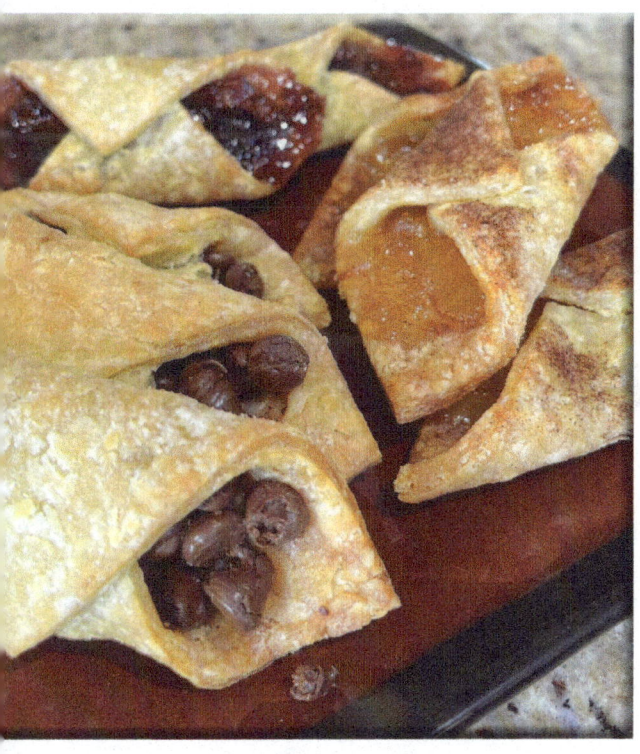

INGREDIENTS
240 g GF flour*
40 g superfine white rice flour*
1 Tbsp sugar (if making a sweet treat)
¾ tsp baking powder
½ tsp kosher salt
16 Tbsp butter (very cold)
40 g sour cream (cold)
80-100 ml ice cold water
1 egg for egg wash

1. Cut butter into Tablespoon slices and place back into refrigerator.
2. Using a food processor, add flour, white flour, sugar, powder, and salt. Pulse a few times.
3. Add butter to the food processor and pulse 4-5 times. You want butter to be marble size.
4. Add sour cream and pulse 2-3 times
5. Slowly add a little water and pulse a few times.
6. Scrape dough on to a floured working surface.
7. Knead with your hands, working into a ball of dough.
8. Wrap dough in plastic wrap and refrigerate for at least one hour.

JōZ Tip: I use Cup 4 Cup™ GF flour and Authentic Foods™ White Rice Flour Superfine. The video for this recipe is super helpful!

JōZ Crescent Rolls

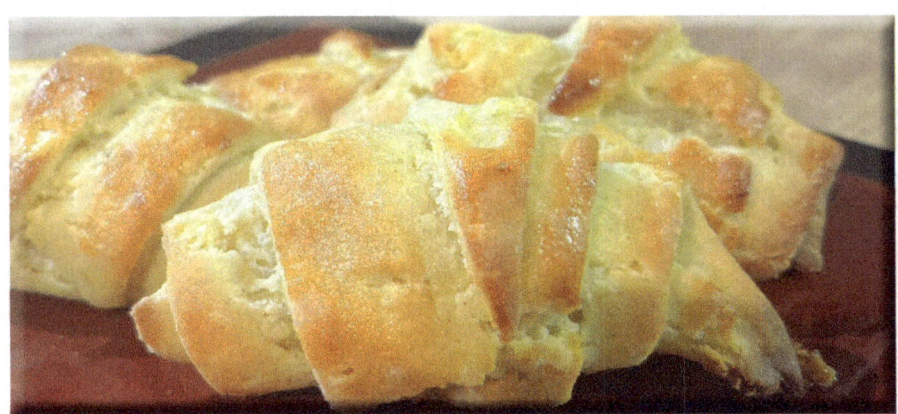

INGREDIENTS

250 g of GF flour*
50 g white rice flour superfine*
1 1/2 Tbsp sugar
1 tsp salt
1 tsp baking powder
½ Tbsp whole milk powder
½ Tbsp psyllium husk powder
½ tsp xanthan gum
1 pkg of instant or fast acting yeast
300 ml milk (warmed)
1 egg
5 Tbsp unsalted butter (melted)

1. Using a large stand mixing bowl, whisk together all dry ingredients.
2. Heat milk until warm and whisk in egg.
3. Pour melted butter into milk. You want milk mixture to be nice and warm but not hot!
4. Using your paddle on your stand mixture, turn on low and slowly add milk mixture into dry mixture. Increase to medium high speed and knead dough for 3 minutes.
5. Taking a rubber spatula sprayed with non-stick spray, scrape dough into a proofing bowl and let rise for at least an hour.
6. Place dough in the refrigerator overnight.
7. When ready to prepare, sprinkle flour liberally on work surface and begin to knead dough.

JōZ Tip: I like to use Cup 4 Cup™ GF flour. Remember practice makes perfect… Don't get discouraged if your first batch isn't successful!! Bread is tricky and it takes time to get the feel. Video does help!!

JōZ Biscuits

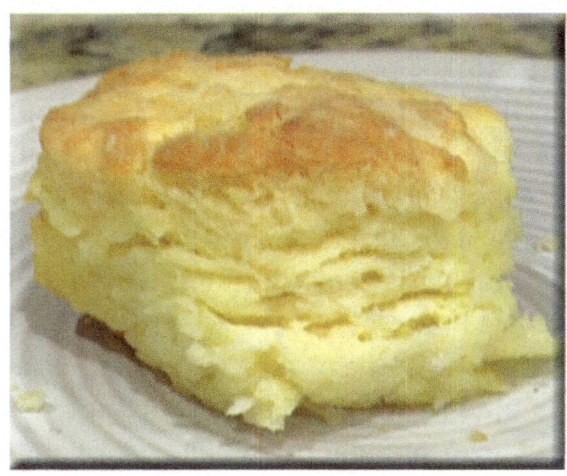

INGREDIENTS

   284 g of GF flour*
   1 1/2 Tbsp Baking powder
   1 tsp baking soda
   ½ tsp salt
   12 Tbsp salted butter* (very cold)
   240 ml buttermilk
   1 egg
   2 Tbsp butter*
   10 in cast iron skillet

1. Preheat oven to 400°**F**.
2. In a large mixing bowl, combine all dry ingredients.
3. Grate or cut in butter.
4. In a small measuring cup, mix buttermilk and egg. Add to dry ingredients.
5. Stir with a large spoon until the dough is combined. **DO NOT OVER STIR**!
6. Place the bowl in the refrigerator.
7. Place 2 Tbsp butter in cast iron skillet and place in oven until butter is completely melted. Remove the skillet from the oven.
8. Sprinkle extra flour on work surface. Working quickly, knead the dough slightly until dough is smooth. Pat dough into a circle about 3/4-1 inch thickness.
9. Using a circle cutter, cut out biscuits and place them in butter then flip over. Repeat until all dough is converted to biscuits.
10. Place in oven and cook for approx. 20-30 mins or until golden brown on top.
11. ENJOY!

JōZ Tip: Watching the Video is very helpful with this recipe. I use Cup 4 Cup ™ Gluten Free flour. **DO NOT** over-knead this dough!! For the dairy free option for this recipe email me at *joz@chefjoz.com*.

For the Love of Gluten Free

JōZ Pie Crust

INGREDIENTS

380 g GF flour*
1 Tbsp sugar
½ tsp baking powder
1 tsp salt
8 Tbsp butter (cold)
   (cut in to ½ Tbsp slices)
65 g butter flavored Crisco™
65 g Spectrum™
120 g – 180 g cold ice water
1 egg (slightly beaten)
1 tsp vinegar
Egg wash and sugar (optional)

1. Mix flour, sugar, salt, and baking powder in a medium size bowl and set aside.
2. Using a stand mixer bowl, add Crisco™ and spectrum and mix on medium speed for 20-30 seconds.
3. Add butter and mix for 10-15 seconds. You want chunks of butter.
4. Add dry ingredients and mix until combined, approximately 20-30 seconds.
5. Add egg and vinegar and start mixer on low and slowly add in water until you get a ball of dough. **DO NOT OVER MIX!**
6. Remove dough from mixing bowl and divide into 2 equal halves. Wrap in cling wrap in shape of a disc and refrigerate for at least one hour.
7. When ready to cook, preheat oven to 375°F.
8. Dust work surface with GF flour and take one disc of dough and roll it out into a circle larger than your pie plate. I like to roll it out on parchment paper, making it easier to transfer into the pie plate.
9. After you have the crust rolled out, place your pie dish on top, upside down, and gently slipping your hand under the parchment paper, flip the dish right side up.
10. Carefully remove parchment paper and form edges to your desired shape.
11. Brush the edges with egg wash and top with a bit of sugar if desired.
12. If blind baking, use a fork and poke a few holes in bottom of pie crust.
13. Bake for 15-17 mins until golden brown.

OR

14. Fill and bake according to your chosen recipe.

JōZ Tip: I use Cup 4 Cup™ GF flour.

IMPORTANT: The video for this recipe is **VERY** helpful!

JōZ Graham Cracker Pie Crust

INGREDIENTS

165 g crushed graham crackers*
2 Tbsp sugar
1 Tbsp dark brown sugar
5-6 Tbsp melted butter

1. Crush graham crackers by using either a zip lock bag and rolling pin, or food processor until fine.
2. Using a medium size mixing bowl, add crushed graham crackers and both sugars. Stir with a fork.
3. Slowly pour in ½ of the melted butter. Stir with fork. Pour in the rest of butter and mix thoroughly with fork. Use as directed in recipe.

JōZ Tip: I either use Schar™ Graham Crackers or Pamela's™ Graham Crackers. Both yield a great result.

JōZ Corn Tortilla

INGREDIENTS

200-240 ml warm/hot water
280 g of corn masa
½ tsp salt
Tortilla Press
large zip lock bag cut into 2 pieces

1. In a large bowl whisk together masa and salt.
2. Slowly add water and work into masa with your hand until a ball forms.
3. Cover with a wet paper towel and set aside for 30 mins.
4. Take dough and pinch off about a golf ball size piece and roll between your palms until a ball forms. Repeat until all dough is gone. Cover with wet paper towel.
5. Start heating your skillet to medium-high heat. I like to use a nonstick just to make it simple.
6. Take 1 side of your zip lock bag and place on bottom of tortilla press. Place a ball of dough on top, then place other piece of zip lock bag on top of dough and press down tortilla press.
7. Gently place tortilla in skillet and cook for about 15 secs and flip over. Cook for about a minute and flip back over. Gently press in the middle of your tortilla and it should start to puff. It is ready. Repeat until all tortillas are made.

JōZ Tip: The video is extremely helpful. If the first attempt is not successful, try again as it may take several attempts to learn the process. Cover tortilla balls with a paper towel to prevent them from drying out.

PRODUCTS I USE IN THIS COOKBOOK

I f you're new to gluten-free cooking, I've listed the products I personally use. At the time of publishing, these products are gluten-free, and I've suggested a few dairy-free options as well. Keep checking back on my website www.chefjoz.com for new product suggestions. Recipes can change over time, so please always double check labels.

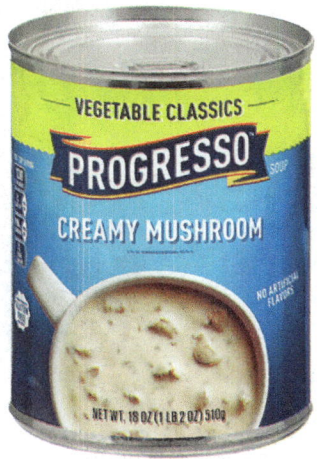
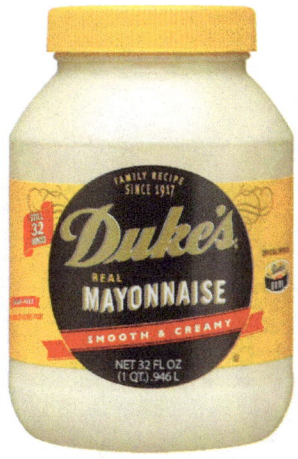
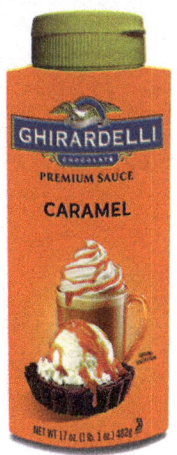
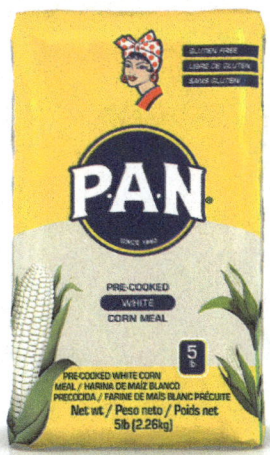

For the Love of Gluten Free

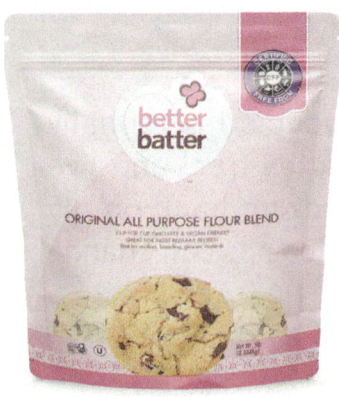
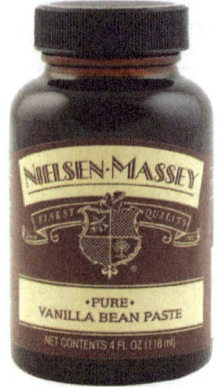
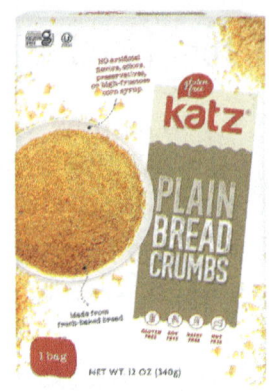
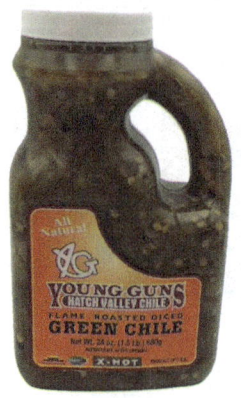
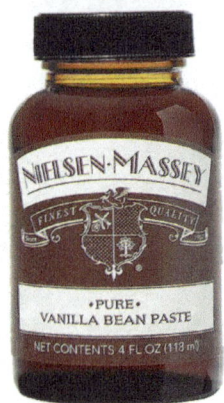
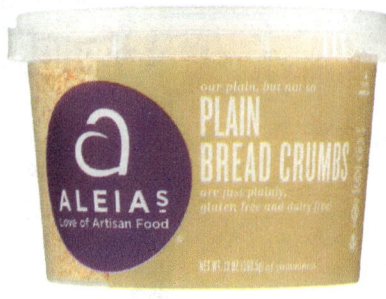
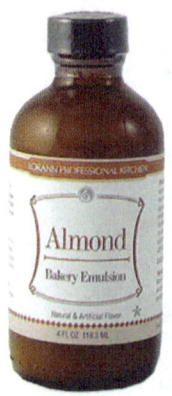
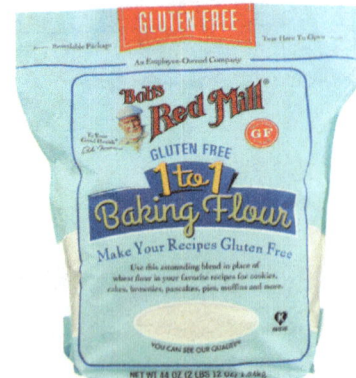
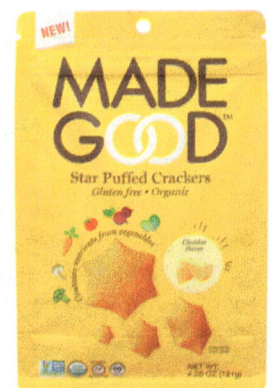
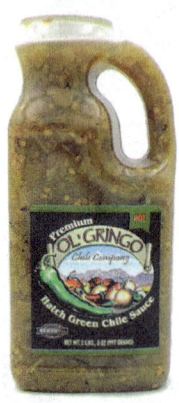
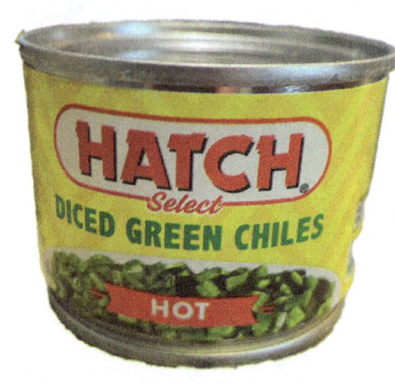
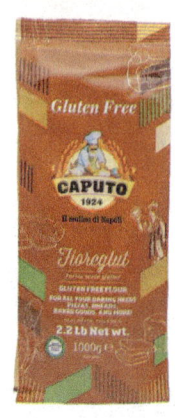

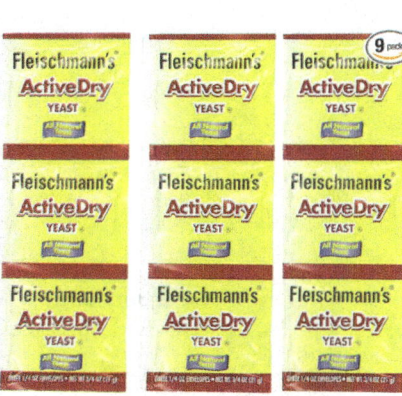 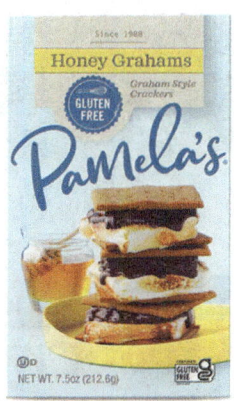 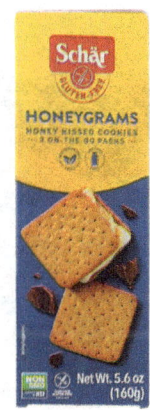
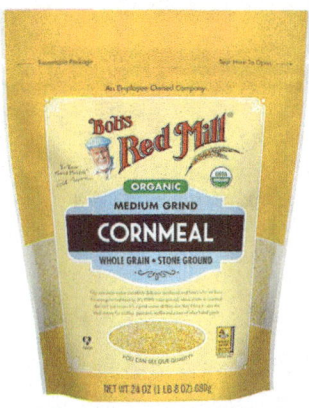 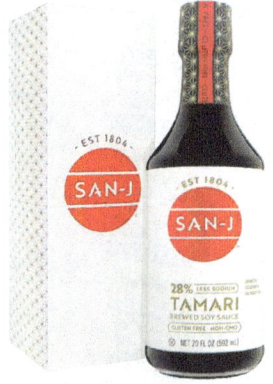 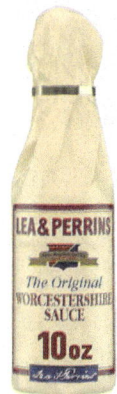
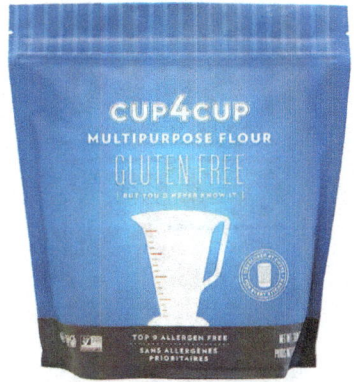 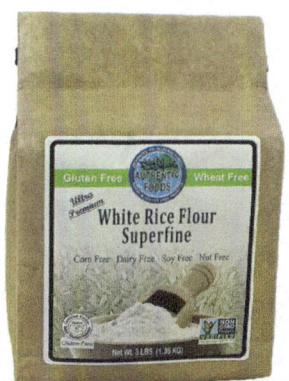 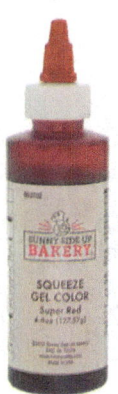
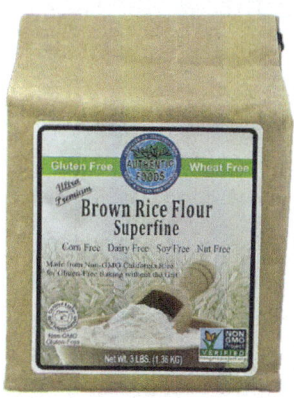 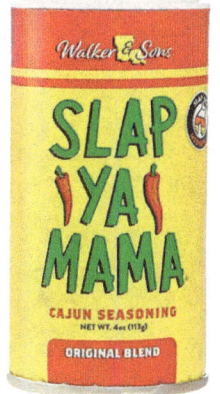 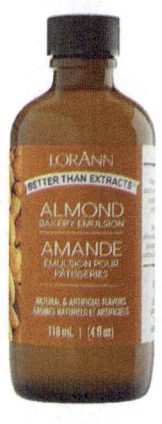

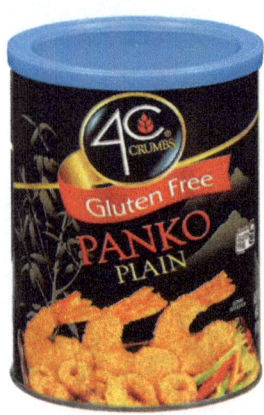 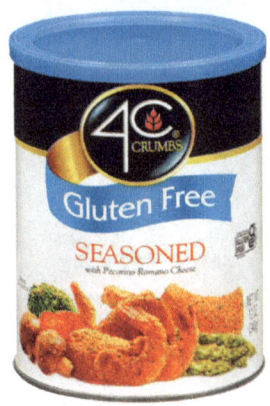 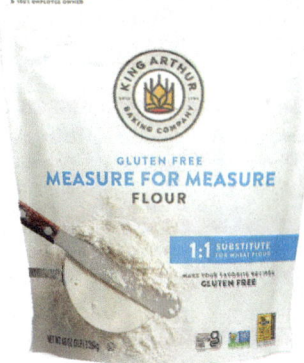
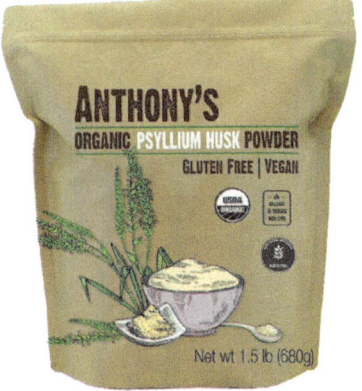 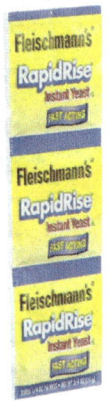 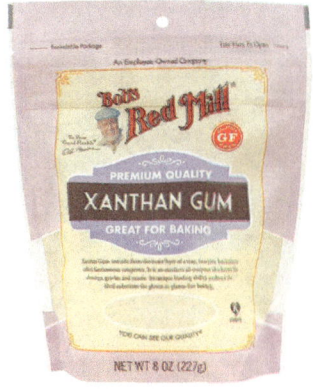
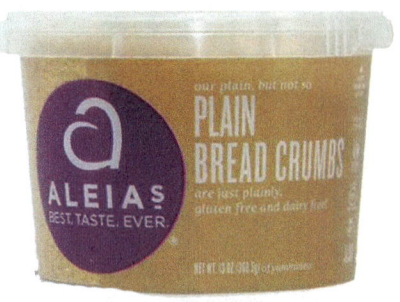 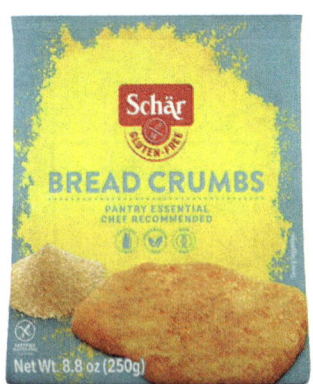 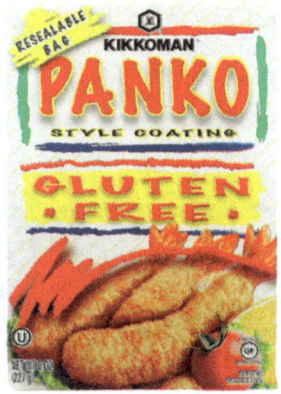
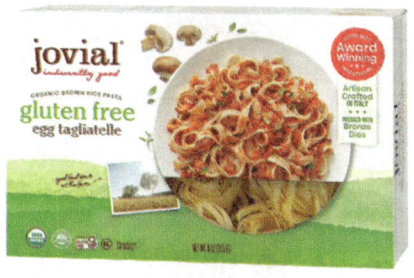 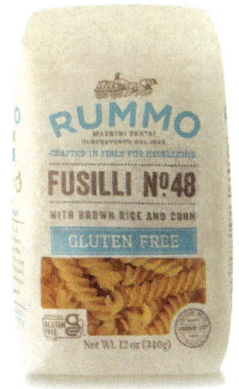 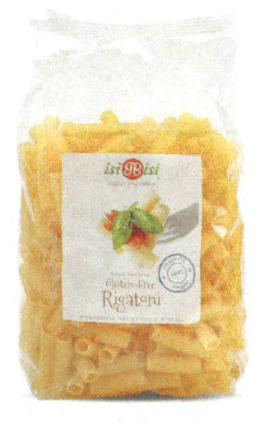

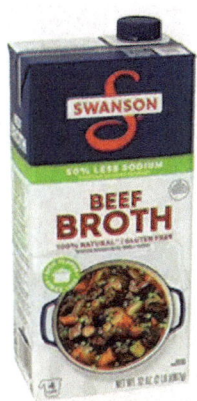
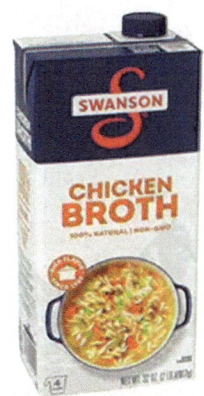
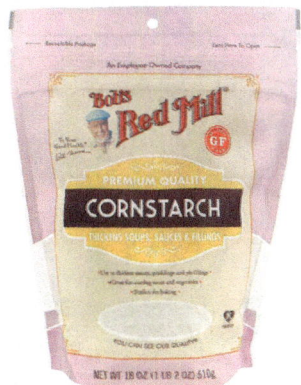
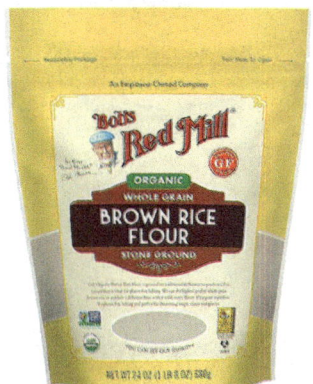
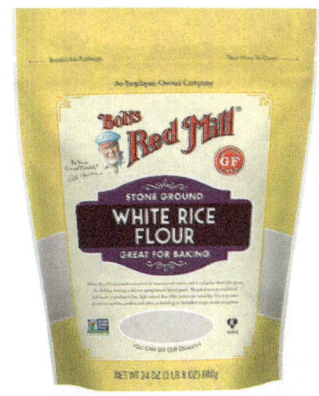
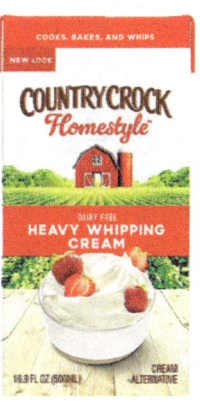
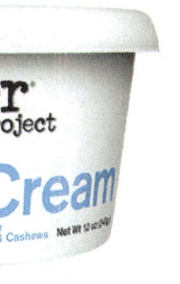
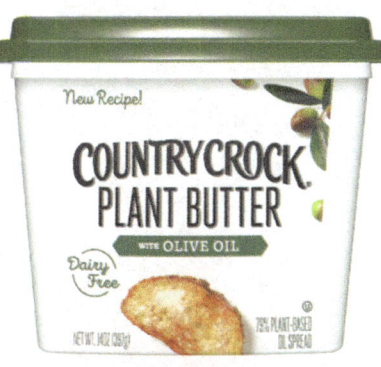
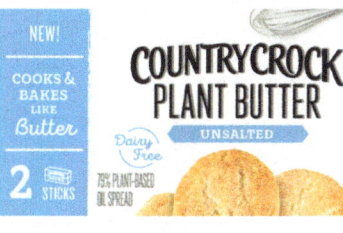
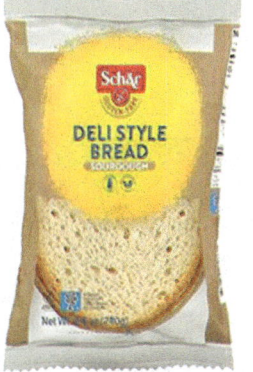
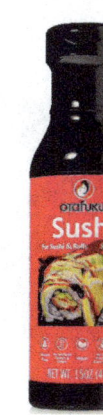
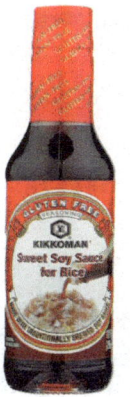

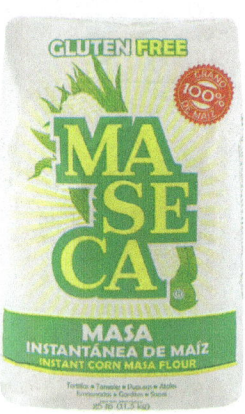 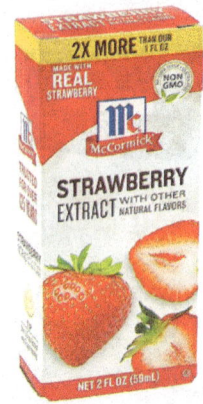 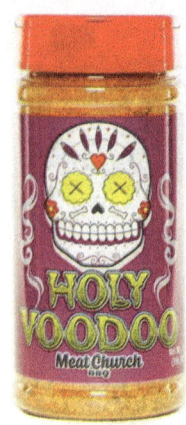
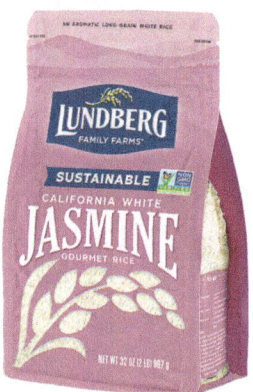 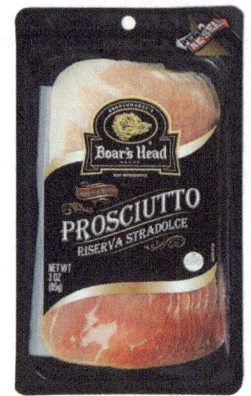 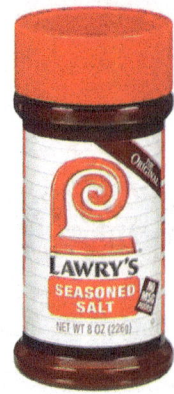
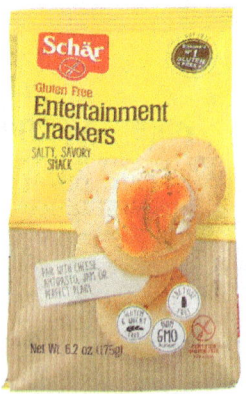 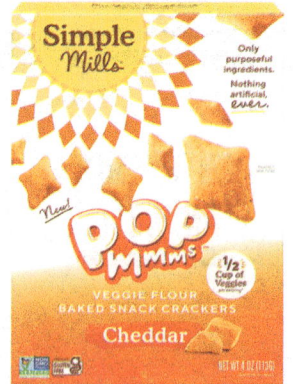 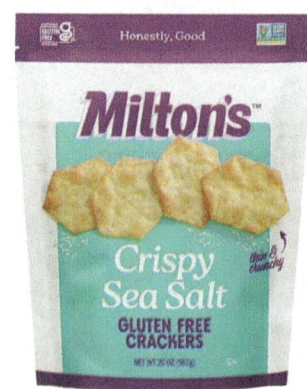
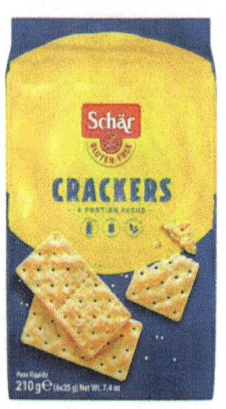 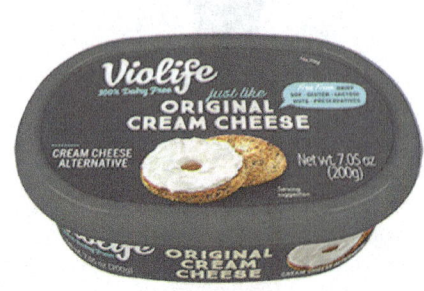 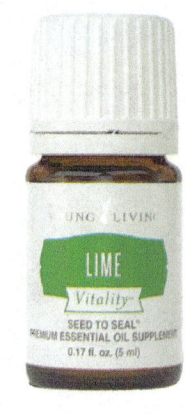

Made in the USA
Coppell, TX
18 January 2026

69140748R00050